Overcoming Common Problems

The Holistic Health Handbook

MARK GREENER

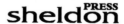

First published in Great Britain in 2013

Sheldon Press
36 Causton Street
London SW1P 4ST
www.sheldonpress.co.uk

British Library Cataloguing-in-Publication Data
A catalogue record for this book is available from the British Library

ISBN 978-1-84709-246-5
eBook ISBN 978-1-84709-247-2

Typeset by Fakenham Prepress Solutions, Fakenham, Norfolk NR21 8NN
First printed in Great Britain by Ashford Colour Press
Subsequently digitally reprinted in Great Britain

Produced on paper from sustainable forests

Mark Greener spent a decade in biomedical research before joining *MIMS Magazine* for GPs in 1989. Since then, he has written on health and biology for magazines worldwide for patients, healthcare professionals and scientists. He is the author of 14 other books, including *Coping with Asthma in Adults* (2011) and *The Heart Attack Survival Guide* (2012), both Sheldon Press. Mark lives with his wife, three children and two cats in a Cambridgeshire village.

Overcoming Common Problems Series

Selected titles

A full list of titles is available from Sheldon Press,
36 Causton Street, London SW1P 4ST and on our website at
www.sheldonpress.co.uk

Breast Cancer: Your treatment choices
Dr Terry Priestman

Coeliac Disease: What you need to know
Alex Gazzola

**Coping Successfully with Chronic Illness:
Your healing plan**
Neville Shone

Coping Successfully with Shyness
Margaret Oakes, Professor Robert Bor
and Dr Carina Eriksen

Coping with Anaemia
Dr Tom Smith

Coping with Drug Problems in the Family
Lucy Jolin

Coping with Early-onset Dementia
Jill Eckersley

Coping with Eating Disorders and Body Image
Christine Craggs-Hinton

Coping with Epilepsy
Dr Pamela Crawford and Fiona Marshall

Coping with Gout
Christine Craggs-Hinton

Coping with Guilt
Dr Windy Dryden

Coping with Liver Disease
Mark Greener

**Coping with Manipulation: When others
blame you for their feelings**
Dr Windy Dryden

Coping with Obsessive Compulsive Disorder
Professor Kevin Gournay, Rachel Piper
and Professor Paul Rogers

Depressive Illness – the Curse of the Strong
Dr Tim Cantopher

The Diabetes Healing Diet
Mark Greener and Christine Craggs-Hinton

Dying for a Drink
Dr Tim Cantopher

**The Empathy Trap: Understanding Antisocial
Personalities**
Dr Jane McGregor and Tim McGregor

**Epilepsy: Complementary and alternative
treatments**
Dr Sallie Baxendale

Fibromyalgia: Your Treatment Guide
Christine Craggs-Hinton

Hay Fever: How to beat it
Dr Paul Carson

The Heart Attack Survival Guide
Mark Greener

How to Beat Worry and Stress
Dr David Delvin

How to Come Out of Your Comfort Zone
Dr Windy Dryden

How to Eat Well When You Have Cancer
Jane Freeman

Living with Complicated Grief
Professor Craig A. White

Living with IBS
Nuno Ferreira and David T. Gillanders

Losing a Parent
Fiona Marshall

**Making Sense of Trauma: How to tell
your story**
Dr Nigel C. Hunt and Dr Sue McHale

Motor Neurone Disease: A family affair
Dr David Oliver

Natural Treatments for Arthritis
Christine Craggs-Hinton

Overcoming Loneliness
Alice Muir

The Panic Workbook
Dr Carina Eriksen, Professor Robert Bor
and Margaret Oakes

**Physical Intelligence: How to take charge
of your weight**
Dr Tom Smith

Reducing Your Risk of Dementia
Dr Tom Smith

**The Self-Esteem Journal: Using a journal
to build self-esteem**
Alison Waines

**Transforming Eight Deadly Emotions
into Healthy Ones**
Dr Windy Dryden

Treating Arthritis: The drug-free way
Margaret Hills and Christine Horner

Treating Arthritis: The supplements guide
Julia Davies

**When Someone You Love Has Depression:
A handbook for family and friends**
Barbara Baker

As always, to Rose, Rory, Ophelia and Yasmin

Contents

Introduction

During the fourteenth century, an Italian priest called Peregrine Laziosi – now the patron saint of cancer sufferers – developed a large bone tumour in his leg. The night before a surgeon planned amputation, St Peregrine prayed intensely. He fell into a trance and saw a vision of Jesus Christ touching his leg. The following morning, the cancer had disappeared. By the time Peregrine died in 1345, at the age of 80 and 20 years after the vision, the malignancy had not recurred.[1]

Today, headlines regularly proclaim that a new treatment is a 'miracle', often based more on public relations hype than scientific evidence. Yet 'real' – medically inexplicable – miracles undoubtedly occur.

While I was writing this book, the International Medical Committee of Lourdes recognized the sixty-eighth miracle among pilgrims to the shrine in south-west France: an Italian nun who started walking after spending years paralysed despite several operations. The committee recognizes miracles only if current science cannot explain the recovery. And such recognition is rare. The committee approved the sixty-seventh miracle in 1999: an 'inexplicable' improvement in a middle-aged Frenchman with multiple sclerosis.

Nevertheless, 'miracles' occur every day. An apparently aggressive cancer that doctors expected to prove rapidly fatal enters remission for several years. Indeed, as we will see, spontaneous remissions of cancer are more common than you might expect. A severely injured person walks after doctors predicted life confined to a wheelchair. People 'turn their lives around' after years struggling against drug or alcohol addiction.

Atheists suggest that just because current medical knowledge cannot explain these 'miracles', you do not need to invoke divine intervention. They point to the rapidly growing scientific evidence highlighting the interactions between your mind, environment and lifestyle that cause, contribute to and help cure disease.

Some theologians counter that God might intervene by using these holistic 'internal healing systems' to give our bodies a 'push' along the path to health. And they point to the numerous scientific studies showing that spirituality and religion are critical for optimal health and well-being. This book looks at how a holistic approach can help you harness these inner forces – whether you feel they derive from a higher power or from biology, or both – to improve your health, well-being and resilience against illness and adversity.

This holistic approach builds on the foundation laid by modern medicines, but also encompasses the psychological, emotional, spiritual and social aspects of illness that may be just as – or even more – important to patients as their symptoms. Yet healthcare professionals often marginalize these intimate interconnections. Indeed, the continuing popularity of complementary treatments partly reflects dissatisfaction with modern medicine's focus on diseases rather than patients. To take one example, between 17 and 78 per cent of people with cancer (depending on the patients studied) use at least one complementary therapy.[2] While acupuncture, naturopathy and biofeedback seem superficially different, they share a common philosophy: better integrating the spiritual, mental, emotional and physical sides of a patient will optimize health and well-being (Figure I.1). In other words, complementary treatments are holistic and place the patient firmly back at the centre of health care.

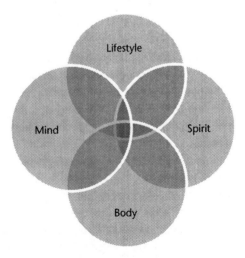

Figure I.1 The holistic view of health

Seeing more and more about less and less

In many ways, doctors' focus on diseases rather than patients – you still hear physicians on a ward discuss 'the heart attack in Bed 6' – is the inevitable consequence of the scientific revolution that saved countless lives and prevented untold suffering. To treat you effectively, doctors need to know 'more and more about less and less', which runs the risk of submerging individual patients in a tsunami of apparently esoteric scientific data.

This wealth of data has largely accumulated since the late nineteenth century as technological advances have allowed scientists to examine tissues in unprecedented detail. As a result, doctors increasingly split ailments that once seemed single diseases into constellations of subtypes based on, for example, genetic variations or abnormal proteins. Pharmacologists (scientists who study drugs) use these insights to create medicines that cure, prevent or manage diseases that terrified our parents and grandparents.

For example, in 1878, physicians from Vienna reported that only 1 in 20 women who underwent surgery for breast cancer lived three years.[3] Modern drugs, radiotherapy and surgery mean that more than three-quarters of women with breast cancer in most Western countries survive at least five years. Even in metastatic breast cancer, where the malignancy has spread to other parts of the body, the number of women aged 60 years or less who survived for five years more than doubled from around 11 per cent of those diagnosed between 1979 and 1984, to about 23 per cent in 2000 to 2004.[4]

Similarly, in 1880, infections and parasitic diseases claimed 33 per cent of lives.[5] Even a scratch could kill. In 1941, Albert Alexander, a policeman in Oxford, developed septicaemia after scratching himself while pruning roses. After becoming the first person to receive penicillin, Alexander improved rapidly. Unfortunately, despite doctors extracting penicillin from his urine, supplies ran out and Alexander relapsed and died.[6]

A few months later, in a Connecticut hospital, Anne Miller was dying from septicaemia after a miscarriage. The morning after her first dose of penicillin, Miller's temperature had dropped from 106°F (41°C) to normal for the first time in a month and she recovered fully: the first life saved by the antibiotic.[7] By 2008, infections and parasitic diseases accounted for just 1 per cent of deaths.[8]

Despite such successes, patients are more than cancerous lumps, raging temperatures or broken bones. Our health responds to our environment. In one study, for example, patients who had a view through their window of a natural setting recovered more rapidly after surgery than a similar group facing a wall.[9] Our health also responds to our social networks. Supportive friends and families, animal companionship and involvement in organized religion all help you stay healthy and live with chronic (long-standing) disease. And health responds to our psychology and spirituality.

The mind in medicine

Healers recognized millennia ago that the mind can produce dramatic physical effects. Writing around 200 AD, the great Graeco-Roman physician Galen noted that depressed women are more susceptible to breast cancer.[10] More recently, some people who witnessed the torture and horrors of the Cambodian killing fields reported fuzzy vision or even blindness, yet doctors could find nothing medically wrong with their eyes.[9] On the other hand, some patients seem able to postpone their death until after an important event. For example, according to *The New York Times*, the city's death rate in the first week of the new millennium rose by 50.8 per cent compared to the final week of 1999.

This book explores how a holistic approach can prevent disease, alleviate symptoms and, occasionally, cure. We'll focus on chronic illnesses, such as heart disease, breathing problems, arthritis and so on. According to Andrew Russell in *The Social Basis of Medicine*, about a third of people in the UK have a chronic illness and a fifth cut down their activities as a result. But rather than focusing on a specific disease, this book looks at the principles that let you control your chronic illness rather than allowing the disease to control you.

Four holistic health principles

Essentially, four principles underpin the holistic approach outlined in this book:

- Maintain an informed, enquiring and collaborative approach with your complementary and conventional healthcare professionals. Several UK surveys show that many patients do not feel as involved in decisions about their care as they would like.[11] Nevertheless, your health and well-being is largely in your hands. However, that *does not* mean you are a victim or that you are responsible for your illness – even if smoking, a poor diet or alcohol abuse contributed to the disease.

- Reduce stress, which contributes to numerous ailments including heart disease, diabetes, arthritis, migraine and ulcerative colitis (inflammation and ulceration of the colon and rectum).[10] Even if stress doesn't cause or exacerbate a disease, you'll feel worse and less able to cope with your illness or problems more generally.
- Make health-promoting lifestyle changes. As we will see, holistic health means tackling four key lifestyle factors that contribute to ill health and developing supportive social networks and partnerships – even with your pets – that bolster your physical, emotional and mental defences.
- Create more efficient, more effective coping strategies by augmenting your spirituality, optimism and resilience. While some of us are naturally more resilient or optimistic than others, it is never too late to bolster your defences. Despite the rise of secularism and atheism, spirituality and religion remain central – to a greater or lesser extent – to the lives of most people in the UK.

In other words, understanding and implementing the principles of holistic health – the interrelationship between lifestyle, mind, body and spirit – improves your chances of a long, rich and fulfilling life.

A word to the wise

This book considers general principles. So, the book *does not* replace advice from your doctor, nurse or pharmacist, who will offer suggestions, support and treatment tailored to your circumstances. You should always see a doctor or nurse if you feel unwell, or think that your disease is getting worse.

While I have included numerous references from medical and scientific studies, it has been impossible to cite all those I referred to. (Apologies to any researchers whose work I have missed.) However, throughout the book I have highlighted certain papers to illustrate key points and themes. Some of these may seem rather erudite if you do not have a medical or biological background. However, do not be put off. You can find a summary by entering the details here: <www.ncbi.nlm.nih.gov/pubmed>. Some full papers are available free online and larger libraries might stock or allow you to access some better-known medical journals.

Contact details for all the organizations mentioned can be found in 'Useful addresses' at the end of the book.

1

The limitations of modern medicine

Better sanitation, clean water, improved nutrition as well as effective and relatively safe vaccinations, medicines and surgical operations mean that we are, in general, healthier than any previous generation. We no longer fear that a scratch could prove fatal, a cough could herald tuberculosis or our children will contract polio while swimming.

And, on average, we live longer than ever. During the seventeenth, eighteenth and much of the nineteenth century, life expectancy was just 30 to 40 years. Government statistics estimate life expectancy for children born between 2008 and 2010 at about 78 years for boys and 82 years for girls. Indeed, 32 per cent of boys and 39 per cent of girls born in 2012 in the UK can expect to celebrate their one hundredth birthday.

However, as mentioned in the introduction, the marginalization of the 'whole patient' is a consequence of the same scientific revolution that transformed our health and longevity. Appreciating modern medicine's limitations helps you understand why you need to take control of your health using a 'holistic' approach and helps you work proactively with your doctors, nurses and other healthcare professionals to optimize your health. But this raises a fundamental question: what is 'health'?

The 'health' enigma

You know when you're under the weather: you feel out of sorts, lethargic, run down. The symptoms of many serious ailments are more obvious: angina's crippling chest pain; flu's raging fever; the discomfort and disability of a broken limb. Yet defining health and disease is more difficult than you might expect. Indeed, Tikkinen and colleagues note that 'disease' 'can be as difficult to define as beauty, truth or love'.[1]

Health – the word derives from old English for 'being sound' (*hoelth*) – isn't simply not being ill. In 1948, the World Health Organization defined health as 'a state of complete physical, mental and social well-being and not merely the absence of disease or infirmity'. The definition underscores that a holistic perspective – encompassing physical, mental and social aspects – is essential for 'health'.

A fundamental problem

Yet this apparently simple definition raises fundamental problems. Most doctors would regard me as reasonably healthy. My blood pressure and other vital signs are normal. Thankfully, I don't currently suffer from any serious diseases. I don't drink excessively or smoke, my diet is reasonably healthy and I exercise fairly regularly. Yet I am constantly niggled by aches, pains and anxieties, and do not have either the time or the money to participate in a 'full social life'. Even on a good day, I'm a long way from being in a state that I would regard as 'complete physical, mental and social well-being'. In other words, I feel dissatisfied with many aspects of my life.

Worryingly, some studies link 'dissatisfaction' with an increased risk of ill health. In one investigation, British civil servants who said they were moderately or highly satisfied with their life were respectively 20 per cent and 26 per cent less likely to develop heart disease (allowing for other risk factors) than those who reported low levels of satisfaction. Indeed, satisfaction with their job, family life, sex life and themselves each reduced the risk of heart disease by around 12 per cent.[2] But how many doctors would regard dissatisfaction with your sex life or job as being 'ill'? Fortunately, as we will see throughout this book, you can change the way you react to life's frustrations.

The impact of culture

To complicate matters further, patients' view of 'complete physical, mental and social well-being' can differ dramatically. A constellation of symptoms that Peter may regard as 'healthy' can leave Paul under the weather. Doctors regularly face the worried well: people who fear a minor ache or pain could be the first sign of a serious illness. On the other hand, some people soldier on with remarkable fortitude despite overwhelming physical or mental handicaps. And our attitudes change as we age. Russell points out that some people – particularly young men – tend to regard health as synonymous with fitness. Older people tend to focus on function: whether they are well enough to take part in their work, hobbies and other activities of everyday life.

Society also strongly influences our definition of 'complete physical, mental and social well-being'. In her fascinating book *The Cure Within*, Anne Harrington notes that Japanese does not even have names for hot flushes (also called hot flashes) or the night sweats experienced by many Western menopausal women. In part, the absence of these symptoms may reflect the fact that female ageing in Japan does not usually carry the same connotations of 'diminished status and worth' as in North America or Europe.

The Western menopausal symptoms illustrate that some people express emotional problems by developing physical symptoms – called somatization. For example, Russell notes, depressed people often complain of vague symptoms, such as aches and pains 'everywhere', tiredness, headaches and dizziness. In English-speaking countries, our bowels bear the brunt of somatization – we're 'sick with fear', have 'the runs' or complain of 'butterflies in the tummy'. Chinese people complain of somatic symptoms in their liver, spleen, heart or kidneys. In Iran and the Punjab, the heart tends to be affected. These symptoms, Russell points out, offer a 'socially acceptable way of indicating emotional distress'.

Napoleon's menstruating men

A striking example of society's impact on symptoms regarded as 'normal' emerged when Napoleon Bonaparte invaded Egypt in 1798. Bonaparte found 'a land of menstruating men', Russell reports. A parasitic worm – schistosomiasis – can invade the bladder. So, infected patients often pass copious amounts of blood in their urine, inspiring Bonaparte's comment. Even today, young boys in rural Egypt sometimes jump in the red urine of infected people to catch a 'disease' they regard as 'normal'.

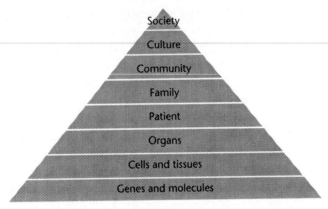

Figure 1.1 A hierarchy of systems influences health and well-being
Source Adapted from Russell

Given the multitude and diversity of factors that influence health and disease, it's not surprising that doctors strip away the social, subjective and emotional elements leaving a core of scientifically identifiable and treatable 'abnormal' biology. Essentially, doctors focus on the levels in Figure 1.1 from 'patient' down. For example, mould in poor housing commonly triggers asthma. Unemployment, debt and economic uncertainty can increase the risk of heart disease and psychiatric illness (page 17). Understandably, doctors tend to alleviate symptoms with drugs rather than try to improve housing or tackle the country's economic woes. (Nevertheless, GPs often refer people to medical social workers to help with benefits and other support services.) But, in some people, tackling the symptoms and not the causes papers over the cracks.

The foundation of modern medicine

Modern medicine is objective, rational and scientific. Doctors use objective signs (e.g. blood pressure and heart rate) and symptoms (e.g. pain or a rash) to diagnose and prescribe. They evaluate a treatment's success based on measurable changes – such as a reduction in blood pressure or cholesterol level, or an obvious improvement in symptoms. Furthermore, as Roberta Bivins notes, a 'potent combination' of laws, regulations, commercial and political interests, culture and public expectations support and sustain this biomedical approach. And the biomedical approach is our most powerful technique to identify the medicines that we rely on. Russell notes that in any 24 hours about half of all adults in the UK probably use a prescribed drug.

Nevertheless, *Exploring Reality*, a thought-provoking and inspiring book by John Polkinghorne (a theoretical physicist who became an Anglican priest), notes that 'science describes only one dimension of the many-layered reality within which we live, restricting itself to the impersonal and general, and bracketing out the personal and unique'. In particular, Polkinghorne adds, the biomedical approach 'has difficulty accounting for psychological, sociological, and spiritual factors that influence most, if not all, illnesses'.[3] Holistic approaches restore the 'personal and unique' by encompassing the psychological, sociological and spiritual factors.

Indeed, Polkinghorne notes, complex systems – such as the human body – generate patterns of effects that studying the individual components would not predict. (The technical term for these patterns – which may include consciousness and life itself – is 'emergent phenomena'.) For example, we know that certain parts of the brain seem to change in alcoholic people. We know the chemical processes that the body uses to break down alcohol. We know that around 50 to 60 per cent of the risk of developing alcoholic liver disease or becoming addicted to drink depends on the genes you inherited from your biological parents.[4] But that's a long way from examining the systems and knowing who will develop a drinking problem, how much they will imbibe on a particular night and their chances of recovery.

And while science is capable of profound insights and stimulating remarkable technological advances, medicine still cannot explain how every effective treatment works. A paper in the prestigious *Archives of Internal Medicine* considered 31 studies – which included almost 18,000 patients – and reported that acupuncture roughly halved the intensity of chronic pain caused by back, neck and shoulder problems, osteoarthritis and headache. Yet, the paper points out, 'there is no accepted mechanism by which [acupuncture] could have persisting effects on chronic pain'.[5]

The diagnostic dilemma

Usually people regard themselves as 'ill' when they develop symptoms – such as pain, the most common reason for a patient to consult his or her doctor. Yet many more people suffer pain than see their doctor. In the UK, at least 50 per cent of those aged 65 years and over, and approximately 60 per cent of people aged over 75 years, report pain or discomfort.[6] Indeed, three-quarters of people in the UK experience at least one symptom in any fortnight. But very few consult their doctors. Symptoms need to cross a biological 'threshold' to develop into a disease. In other words, Russell notes, illness is the 'subjective, psychological experience' – the mental and physical symptoms. You become 'sick' when society recognizes your illness, such as a doctor diagnosing a disease or you taking time off from your work.

But the biological changes that cause disease may have harmed your body – perhaps irreparably – by the time symptoms emerge and you decide to see your doctor. So, doctors increasingly use sophisticated technology to pinpoint early abnormalities before a disease develops, such as malignancies that are sufficiently small and localized to allow a cure. Similarly, scanning the density of your bone helps detect whether you are vulnerable to an osteoporotic (brittle-bone disease) fracture. Measuring blood pressure or cholesterol helps determine how likely you are to have a heart attack or stroke.

However, many of these early abnormalities never develop sufficiently to cause symptoms. As a result, you may be treated – and experience side effects – for a disease you would have never developed. For example, breast cancer becomes more common as women get older. As a result, many women die of other causes before the cancer brings about symptoms. Researchers analysing the Norwegian mammography (breast scan) programme found that between 15 per cent and 25 per cent of breast cancers would not have produced problems during the patient's life.[7] These women potentially underwent surgery, radiotherapy and treatment with toxic drugs for a cancer that would not have emerged. Nevertheless, as doctors cannot tell who will develop clinical cancer, most believe the benefits of mammography outweigh the risks. On the other hand, up to 40 per cent of people undergoing imaging of their abdomen, pelvis, chest, head and neck show 'abnormalities' other than those the scan aimed to detect.[8] So, discuss the risks and benefits of treating any incidental findings with your doctor.

Nevertheless, doctors often cannot detect an unambiguous abnormality or specific symptoms. So they diagnose by referring to 'agreed' diagnostic criteria. However, if doctors change the definition, the number of affected people also alters. For example, when should we treat grief with antidepressants (page 42)? When does an eye for detail become obsessive-compulsive disorder? What level of blood pressure carries sufficient risk of a stroke to warrant treatment? Too strict a definition denies people the help they need. Too liberal a definition means that unnecessary treatment will cause side effects. It's a judgement call, which is why you should discuss the risks and benefits with your doctor.

When healing harms

More than 500 years ago, Philippus Aureolus Theophrastus Bombastus von Hohenheim (1493–1541) – better known as Paracelsus – observed that 'The dose makes the poison.' For example, even mild dehydration can cause a variety of unpleasant symptoms (page 60). However, drinking too much water can kill: in 2007, a woman died after drinking six litres of water in three hours. Botulinum toxin, produced by a bacterium, is one of the most toxic poisons; however, minuscule doses can alleviate muscle spasms and spasticity and reduce the appearance of wrinkles.

Even drugs in family medicine boxes can cause potentially fatal side effects. For example, in some cases less than 4 g paracetamol a day can damage the liver.[9] Indeed, in 2010, paracetamol poisoning contributed to 199 deaths – in other words, the death certificate mentions the painkiller. That's more than the number who died from cocaine (mentioned on 144 death certificates), amphetamines (56) or cannabis (11).

So, modern medicine depends on balancing a treatment's risks and benefits for each patient. For example, doctors and patients typically accept a higher risk of serious side effects (also called adverse events) for a drug that could cure a fatal cancer. They are less likely to accept even a miniscule risk for vaccines or contraceptives given to otherwise healthy people. Furthermore, the acceptable risk varies between patients. For example, you may agree to take a more potent painkiller for osteoarthritis – and accept the higher risk of side effects – if you want to ramble across the countryside than if you're happy just wandering around the local shopping centre.

Nevertheless, many people suffer unnecessary adverse events. Indeed, side effects from prescription medicines contribute to around 1 in 15 hospital admissions. The adverse event led directly to the admission in four of five cases, and approximately 1 in 50 of those admitted with a side effect died as a direct result. Tragically, better use of the medicines could have avoided almost three-quarters (72 per cent) of these adverse events.[10] So, speak to your GP, nurse or pharmacist if you feel you are developing side effects or you are worried about adverse events. But never stop a drug or reduce the dose without speaking to a doctor first.

Complementary risks

Complementary therapies are, generally, less biologically active than conventional medicines – but they can still cause serious adverse events. Just because a treatment is natural does not necessarily make it safe. For example, kava kava *(Piper methysticum)* derives its name from the Polynesian word *awa*, meaning bitter. Traditional preparations made from the shrub produce mild intoxication and are central to many ceremonial and social gatherings in Pacific Island culture. Traditional healers used kava kava to treat numerous diseases including gonorrhoea, syphilis, cystitis and insomnia. In Europe, herbalists used kava kava to treat anxiety. Clinical trials suggest that it works.[11]

At recommended therapeutic doses, kava kava can cause side effects such as skin redness, headache and liver damage.[11] Indeed, by 2006, the Food Standards Agency had received 110 reports over several years in which kava kava possibly caused liver damage. Eleven patients received liver transplants and nine died. Kava kava is banned in the UK. (Nevertheless, in 2006 *alone* paracetamol contributed to 309 deaths – and remains available in supermarkets.) Kava kava underlines the importance of remaining vigilant for side effects with conventional and complementary medicines.

Other mainstays of modern medicine can also cause adverse events. In 1895, the German scientist Wilhelm Conrad Röentgen accidentally discovered X-rays while experimenting with vacuum tubes. A week later, Röentgen took the first radiograph: of his wife's hand, showing her bones and wedding ring. X-rays revolutionized diagnosis and offered a new treatment for many cancers. However, experimenters soon recognized that X-rays cause burns and skin reactions. Then, in 1902, an X-ray technician developed a cancer on his hand, which killed him four years later.[12] Today, we know that X-rays increase the risk of cancer. However, the benefits usually outweigh the relatively small risks.

In some cases, the harm isn't as obvious. For instance, 80 per cent of women referred for further tests after mammograms did not have breast cancer. These 'false positives' can cause considerable distress, anxiety and expense. Such problems notwithstanding, modern medicine saves countless lives and prevents untold suffering. But you need to balance the risks and benefits.

Bridging the gap

We've seen that doctors tend to take a scientific view of illness, while patients often have a personal holistic perspective.[3] Such differences can cause communication problems. For example, some people prefer a 'paternalistic' doctor. They want the doctor to 'tell' them the diagnosis and treatment. Others expect doctors to respect and acknowledge their viewpoint, even if it conflicts with the doctor's perspective, and to reach a 'negotiated' deci-sion. Others prefer a 'consumerist' approach where patients' rather than doctors' views predominate – as in a commercial transaction.

Communication problems can arise when a paternalistic doctor imposes treatment on a patient who needs to negotiate, or vice versa, or if the doctor dismisses a deeply held view about an alterna-tive treatment, or social or religious factors. For example, the Koran exempts people with serious illness from fasting. Nevertheless, many Muslims with diabetes want to fast, which leaves them at risk of potentially dangerous falls in their blood glucose levels (hypogly-caemic attacks). In many cases, changing management can allow patients with diabetes to fast safely.[13] However, doctors need to be sensitive to the importance that many Muslims attach to the fast and patients have to 'trust' their physician to take their concerns seriously.

The problem of pain

Some symptoms – such as pain, depression or anxiety – are inherently subjective, which contributes to the communication gap and can lead medical staff to underestimate your suffering. Pain is particularly personal. Occasionally, people are born without the ability to feel pain and can handle burning coals, stab knives into their arms and drive spikes through their hands without flinching. On the other hand, some patients born without arms or legs endure phantom pain in a limb that never developed. Most of us are between these extremes. But for any particular stimulus (such as fixed pressure or immersing a hand in water at a set temperature), our perception of pain severity as well as our emotional, biological and behavioural responses can vary dramatically.

Pain's deeply personal nature means that healthcare professionals may not fully appreciate patients' suffering. For example, nurses underestimated pain severity, emotional impact and suffering experienced by people undergoing surgery.[14] In another study, nurses' perception of the pain experienced by children was significantly lower than the assessments made by parents and children. Interestingly, parents' and children's scores tended to agree.[15]

Keeping a diary

Keeping a diary of your pain, depression, anxiety or any other subjective symptom can help you explain your suffering to your doctor:

- Even if there is nothing to report, complete the diary each day for a couple of weeks (or two to three months if symptoms emerge less commonly, such as migraines or anxiety around the time of your period). In some cases, your doctor might offer a diary for your condition and there are apps for smart phones and computers.
- Consider ranking your symptoms on a scale of 1–5, where 1 is no pain (or the absence of the symptom) and 5 the most severe imaginable.
- Note any possible triggers (such as what you were doing when the symptom flared) and track the response to treatment. You can also note the impact on your quality of life and day-to-day activities.

- You could note, and reflect on, how you feel physically, emotionally and spiritually. These notes – which are for your eyes only – may help you understand your illness, come to terms with the disease and imagine your alternatives.

> **Reading for your health**
>
> You may find that reading about how other people overcame adversity helps. As we'll see later (page 86), reading can help you act as your own therapist. Reading fiction and nonfiction helps you explore and understand your problems and focus on something other than your issues. Some areas hold formal 'bibliotherapy' groups. Ask your local library if there is a group near you.

The communication checklist

Taking responsibility for your holistic health means asking questions, which your doctor, nurse and pharmacist will be happy to answer. Do not be afraid to ask: most healthcare professionals welcome full discussions. And make sure you let your doctor know the full range and severity of your symptoms and problems. Doctors base about 80 per cent of diagnoses on what patients reveal. However, Russell comments that when questioned after seeing their GP, about 60 per cent of patients had not disclosed some of their symptoms during the consultation, because, for example, they felt asking was inappropriate, or they feared a bad reaction, or felt hurried. Your doctor can't diagnose and treat you appropriately without a full picture.

On the other hand, doctors can become 'fixed' on one problem and ignore other explanations – so-called diagnostic overshadowing. A doctor might attribute aches and pains in an obese person to excess weight, when the discomfort arises from, for instance, gall bladder disease, arthritis or fibromyalgia. A person with depression can develop chest or bowel symptoms that a doctor may 'dismiss' as somatization (page 3). The best way to overcome diagnostic overshadowing is to give the doctor a full picture and insist that you are sure that your chronic diseases do not cause the problem.

To aid your conversations, learn all you can about the disease and treatment options from patient groups, friends and relatives.

(Unless they are medically qualified, check their advice. People can, with the best will in the world, offer misleading or out-of-date advice.) You will almost certainly surf around the internet. Although an invaluable resource, sites may be inaccurate or misleading, or promote a commercial or vested interest. So, it's a good idea to check the 'about us' pages. For instance, some internet sites promote AIDS denial – the now discredited claim that HIV does not cause AIDS – or the idea that pharmaceutical companies are suppressing a single cure for cancer. (A single cure for cancer is probably impossible. Cancer is, in reality, more than two hundred different diseases that vary depending on the organ, stage and underlying molecular abnormalities. In any case, modern treatments already cure some malignancies.) Try to ensure the site is reputable, such as one recommended by a patient group or your doctor.

As we've seen, the decision to use a drug depends on the balance of risks and benefits. Whenever your doctor prescribes a new drug, suggests changing the dose or advocates an operation, make sure that you fully understand the hazards and the expected benefits. Just discussing your fears, concerns and ambitions can alleviate the emotional and psychological burden and can make you feel better. You might want to take a pad and pen into the consultation – or photocopy the checklist in Table 1.1.

Generic prescribing

Your pharmacist may dispense unbranded 'generic' medicines, which are usually much cheaper than brands. (The NHS invests the money saved to meet other priorities.) Each brand and generic meets stringent quality criteria – generics are not inferior – and, in most cases, switching does not undermine effectiveness or trigger side effects. However, there are a few exceptions, such as certain drugs for epilepsy, asthma and raised blood pressure. So, if you feel anything unusual or think that the control of your symptoms has worsened, contact your GP.

Table 1.1 The communication checklist

What is the name of the drug or the procedure?

Why is this the best treatment for me?

What are the side effects or complications?

How often or when should I take the medicine?

What should I do if I miss a dose?

What should I do if I accidentally take another dose too soon?

Is there any risk of interactions?

How do I know if the drug is working? How do I know if the operation has worked?

When should I return for review?

- *What is the name of the drug or the procedure?* You should know the medical name of the procedure (to help you look it up) or the drug's brand and scientific ('generic') names. For example, sildenafil is the generic name for the brand Viagra. A medicine can have several brand names and different packaging, but the generic name remains the same. You need to look up both names.
- *Why is this the best treatment for me?* What are the risks and benefits? Will the treatment cure or alleviate symptoms? How do the risks and benefits compare to the alternative treatments? The numbers needed to treat and harm (see the box on page 14 could help you balance the risks and benefits. If your doctor suggests an operation, you might like to know how the success and complication rates in that hospital or for that surgeon compare to the national average. Remember, however, that some better surgeons might seem statistically less successful because they treat more difficult cases.
- *What are the side effects or complications?* Read the patient information leaflet included in the package or online (<www.medicines.org.uk/emc/>) and speak to your doctor, nurse or pharmacist if you have concerns or questions. Ask whether there are any symptoms to watch for that might indicate side effects or complications. If you are undergoing an operation, ask when you can take part in activities such as driving, returning to work and exercise.

- *How often or when should I take the medicine?* Make sure you know what to do if you miss a dose or accidentally take another dose too soon. If you only need to use a drug occasionally, make sure your stocks at home are in date. There are some tips to help you stick to treatment later in this chapter.
- *Is there any risk of interactions?* Some drugs interact with other medicines, foods, complementary therapies and drugs bought 'over the counter' from pharmacists and supermarkets. Read the patient information leaflet and tell your doctor and pharmacist if you are taking other medicines.
- *How do I know if the drug is working?* Some risk factors – such as high blood pressure or raised cholesterol – for potentially life-threatening diseases do not generally cause symptoms and, as a result, need regular monitoring. So, ask when and how often you should return for a check-up. In some cases, a nurse or pharmacist may perform these routine checks. Regular review also offers the opportunity to ensure that, if you have taken a drug for a while, you still need it. However, never stop a drug or change the dose without speaking to your healthcare professional first.

Numbers needed to treat and harm

Not everyone benefits from or experiences side effects with a particular medicine. The drug's 'number needed to treat' (NNT) and 'number needed to harm' (NNH) can help you balance risks and benefits. The NNT represents how many patients would need treatment with a drug, operation or another intervention to produce a particular benefit. Broadly, NNTs of 2.3, 3.6 and 8.9 correspond to 'large', 'medium' and 'small' benefits respectively.[16] In other words, a highly effective drug would benefit one person for about every two treated. The other patient would not benefit, but could still develop side effects. A less effective drug would benefit one person for every nine or so treated. In other words, eight patients would not benefit, but would still be at risk of adverse events. NNH represents how many patients would need treatment to produce one or more adverse events. A NNH of three means that a third of patients develop side effects.

Sticking to treatment

As mentioned earlier, a biological abnormality may need to be relatively advanced before symptoms emerge. A heart attack may be the first sign that you have diabetes, for example, or dangerously high blood pressure (hypertension). This lack of symptoms means that you may not feel any improvement when you take your medicines. However, side effects might mean you feel worse – which leads some people to stop taking potentially life-saving medicines or reduce the dose or frequency (called non-adherence, non-compliance or non-concordance). If you feel that you are developing side effects, speak to your GP: there is usually an alternative.

In other cases, you might need treatment for several diseases. For example, you may take a couple of drugs to lower blood pressure (often one medicine is not enough), another to tackle elevated cholesterol, another for osteoarthritis in your knee and an antidepressant. Taking several drugs (polypharmacy) is especially common among elderly people. One study of people with diabetes living in nursing homes in Coventry found that 84 per cent took at least four medicines.[17] Another study included 467 people aged 75 years of age or over attending an emergency department at a London hospital. Almost 54 per cent took at least four medicines and about 11 per cent took ten or more drugs. Four patients took at least 15 medicines.[18] Apart from the risk that the drugs will interact, some people get confused, which undermines compliance.

Trouble taking your medicines?

Do not be embarrassed to admit to your GP, nurse or pharmacist that you're confused or can't follow the instructions. People may misunderstand treatment instructions – especially if they need to take several drugs – or may simply forget. Your GP and pharmacist can help by offering adherence aids (such as a box that allows you to organize your tablets day by day). People with arthritis or other physical disabilities may experience difficulties opening packaging or swallowing medication. Pharmacists may be able to suggest alternative packaging, such as avoiding 'child-resistant' pill bottles, or dosing forms including liquid versions of the medicine.

This combination of deliberate and accidental non-adherence means that many people do not take their drugs as prescribed. As a rule of thumb, you need to take at least four of every five doses to benefit from a medicine.[19] However:

- Just over a third of patients are non-adherent to oral drugs that treat diabetes.[20]
- One in 250 patients with a high risk of heart disease suffers a non-fatal heart attack after stopping aspirin.[21] (Aspirin reduces the risk of a blood clot inside the blood vessels supplying the heart. This clot causes most heart attacks.)
- Patients who took, on average, 96 per cent of their antihypertensive doses (which lower blood pressure) were 10 per cent less likely to develop coronary artery disease (which causes heart attacks) than those taking, on average, 59 per cent.[22]
- Patients who took at least 80 per cent of their statins (which lower cholesterol levels) were after one year 18 per cent less likely to develop cardiovascular disease than those who took less than 20 per cent.[22]

In other words, taking your medicines as suggested by your doctor is an important element of your holistic health. But as we'll see in the rest of book, it's not the whole story.

2

The mind in medicine

While doctors generally focus their diagnostic and therapeutic skills on diseased tissue or organs – often isolated from the rest of the body, let alone from the mind and spirit – our mental state profoundly affects our bodies. For instance, it might seem like a joke from *Carry on Doctor*, but Japanese researchers found that when women measured the blood pressure of men aged between 18 and 20 years, readings were, on average, 5 mmHg higher than when men made the recording. Almost 11 per cent of young men showed readings sufficient high to diagnose a type of hypertension when women measured blood pressure compared with 4 per cent when men took the readings. However, the sex of the person measuring did not influence blood pressure or heart rate in females of the same age. The researchers called the phenomenon 'white skirt hypertension'.[1]

Austerity and ill health

Unfortunately, the link between the mind and the body is not always amusing. For example, unemployment is a major cause of stress (see page 21), which can trigger heart disease. Indeed, researchers found that the risk of suffering a heart attack increased by 35 per cent among unemployed people, especially during the first year on the dole, compared to those in work. The risk of suffering a heart attack rose as the number of job losses increased: 22 per cent for one loss; 27 per cent for two; 52 per cent for three; and 63 per cent for at least four job losses. Indeed, the increased risk of suffering a heart attack linked to unemployment was similar to other major risk factors, including smoking (44 per cent increase), diabetes (51 per cent) and hypertension (62 per cent).[2] Other studies show that deaths from diseases of the heart and blood vessels (cardiovascular) disease, abnormal heart rhythms (arrhythmias) and heart attacks rise immediately after disasters such as earthquakes and terrorist attacks.[3]

In addition, economic problems – such as debt or unemployment – cause mental health issues. However, some people are in debt or are unemployed because of mental health problems. For example:

- An analysis of more than 300 papers suggested that 34 per cent of unemployed people endure psychological problems, more than twice the rate among the employed (16 per cent).[4]
- Debt increases the risk of common mental disorders almost three-fold, according to a study of 7,461 adults interviewed in England during 2007. Of the 8.5 per cent who reported being in debt, 38.0 per cent had at least one common mental disorder compared to 13.9 per cent of those without debt. For instance, debt increased the risk of social and other phobias almost four-fold and panic disorder more than three-fold. People in debt were also around twice as likely to have obsessive-compulsive disorder, depression and generalized anxiety.[5]
- The Asian economic crisis in the late 1990s promoted a sharp increase in suicide rates among Japanese and Hong Kong men (by 39 per cent and 44 per cent respectively). A study of 26 EU countries between 1970 and 2007 found that each 1 per cent increase in unemployment increased suicide rates among people younger than 65 years by 0.79 per cent.[4]

Addictions increase the pressure

Alcohol, drug and gambling problems exacerbate the link between debt and mental health. People in debt who were not dependent on alcohol or drugs were almost three times more likely to develop a common mental disorder. Alcohol and drug dependence increased the risk about seven- and eight-fold respectively. People in debt who did not have a gambling problem were approximately three times more likely to develop a common mental disorder. A gambling problem increased the risk almost seven-fold.[5]

Can your personality make you ill?

In the early 1950s, the American cardiologist Meyer Friedman wondered why the seats in the waiting room needed regular repair. The upholsterer commented that the wear pattern suggested that

Table 2.1 Characteristics of type A and type B personality

Type A	Type B
Highly competitive	Non-competitive
Impatient	Unhurried
Goal-orientated	Relaxed
Aggressive	Passive
Restless, rapid movements	More relaxed movements
Not a good listener	Good listener
Fast talker	Talks at a reasonable speed

patients sat on the edge of their seats and clutched the armrests – almost as if they were anxious to leave as soon as possible.

So Friedman and his colleague Ray Rosenman characterized the differences between people who developed heart problems and those who didn't. People Friedman and Rosenman described as 'type A personalities' tend be competitive, impatient, aggressive, ambitious and continually on the go – and are much more prone to high blood pressure and heart disease than the more 'laid back' type B people (see Table 2.1). Higher levels of stress-related hormones (see page 24) in people with type A personalities probably contribute to the increased risk of heart disease.

Since Friedman and Rosenman's pioneering experiments, other studies have linked personality types with certain diseases. For example:

- Patients who scored highly on questionnaires measuring neuroticism (a personality trait linked to stress) were around three times more likely to develop asthma than those with low scores.[6]
- Type C patients tend to repress anger, and cannot effectively recognize or communicate negative emotions. Often they feel hopeless and useless, and lack self-control when stressed. Some studies suggest that women with type C personalities may be especially prone to developing breast cancer.[7]
- People with type D personalities (D for 'distressed') experience persistent negative emotions, pessimism and social inhibition (e.g. intense shyness and introspection). Fear of disapproval means that they do not share their negative emotions. In one

study, people with type D personalities were three times more likely to need angioplasty (an operation that opens blood vessels blocked by heart disease) or by-pass surgery, or to suffer problems such as heart failure, heart transplantation, heart attacks and death from cardiovascular disease.[8]

This link does not mean that cancer, heart attack or any disease for that matter results from a 'weak' personality. Personality is one of a plethora of factors that influence risk, in the same way as alcohol or eating a high-fat diet. You can take steps to reduce the overall impact on your health by addressing the other risk factors – smoking is a much more potent carcinogen than personality. Cognitive behavioural therapy (page 84), mindfulness (page 85), spirituality (Chapter 3) or counselling (page 84) can help you develop more appropriate coping strategies and bolster your resilience (Chapter 7). Your personality is not set in stone.

The sick role

Your personality changes – to a certain extent – when you admit you are ill: you adopt a 'sick role'. In the 1950s, the American sociologist Talcott Parsons suggested that this sick role carries certain expectations, rights and obligations. When you are sick, you may avoid your normal work and family responsibilities. However, you are under the obligation to seek medical treatment and comply with doctor's orders. The doctor legitimizes the sickness. The medical and social benefits associated with the sick role help you recover more rapidly.

Despite the short-term benefits, it is important not to become caught in a sick role. In the 1920s, doctors recognized that some patients deliberately or subconsciously triggered severe diabetic attacks to avoid difficult situations at home by 'escaping' into hospital.[9] A person may suffer asthma symptoms before having to make a presentation at work. Arthritis may flare before a visit to the mother-in-law. The person experiencing these 'psychosomatic' symptoms is not pretending. Rather, it's an unconscious (somatic) expression of emotional distress. Keeping a diary about your illness helps you identify whether you might have a subconscious escape route from a stressful situation – and then you can find solutions.

What is stress?

Despite its reputation, stress isn't always bad. You need a certain amount of stress to crawl out of bed in the morning. Many actors, musicians and people making presentations welcome 'stage fright': the heightened arousal enhances their performance. Horror film aficionados delight in the frisson of fear. In other words, 'stress' describes our level of arousal.

As we become more aroused, our sympathetic nervous system (see page 23) becomes more active, glands release hormones, we mobilize energy and our mental abilities sharpen. That's why too little stress can lead to boredom, apathy and poor concentration. In other words, there is a 'n-shaped' link between stress and performance (see Figure 2.1).

However, too many of us have too much of a good thing. Over-arousal – what most people mean by 'stress' – undermines performance. You feel stressed when the demands on you increase your arousal to a point that outstrips your resources, strengths and time. Your body will begin to tell you that you are overdoing it.

When physical or psychological symptoms emerge, when you drink excessively, when your relationships suffer, it is probably time you took stock and recharged your batteries. Many people do not heed their body's advice: they ignore the warning signs and are at risk of physical and mental illness. For example:

• Some American soldiers who died on Omaha Beach, arguably the most fiercely fought bridgehead in the D-Day landings, showed only superficial flesh wounds. They probably died from terror.[10]

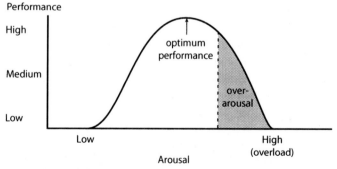

Figure 2.1 The n-shaped link between stress and performance

- In one study, the risk of stillbirth was 18 per cent higher among people whose first-degree relative died (often intensely stressful) in the year before or during the pregnancy.[11]
- Bottling-up stress-related tension is a risk factor for many ailments including heart disease, diabetes, arthritis, migraine and ulcerative colitis.[12]
- Divorce or the end of a 'life partnership' – highly stressful events – approximately doubled the likelihood of developing asthma.[6]
- An Australian study found that work-related stress increased the risk of depression or anxiety by 54 per cent. Personal stress increased the risk of circulatory diseases by 72 per cent, depression or anxiety by 70 per cent and type 2 diabetes (the type that usually emerges in middle age) by 47 per cent. Family-related stress increased the likelihood of the onset of heart and circulatory diseases by 32 per cent.[13]

On the other hand, bolstering your resilience (Chapter 7) and taking a holistic approach to health can move you back towards peak performance. And the various stressors add up. So, while tackling a persistent, stress-inducing problem at work will not necessarily directly improve your asthma, heart disease or cancer, your improved performance will probably mean you feel better.

Inside your nervous system

Nerves connect every part of your body to your brain: you know almost immediately when you stub your big toe, touch a hot pan or hit your thumb with a hammer. In turn, the brain passes signals along these nerves to ensure your body meets the demands of the environment, such as increasing your heartbeat, respiration rate and endurance when you need to run for the train.

Your brain and spinal cord make up your central nervous system (CNS). Biologists divide the nerves outside the CNS – the peripheral nervous system – into two parts:

- The 'somatic' or 'voluntary' nervous system allows us to choose an action. Your voluntary nervous system told your muscles to turn the pages of this book.

- The 'autonomic' or 'involuntary' nervous system maintains our body's essential functions – such as breathing and heartbeat – without conscious control, such as while we're asleep.

It's easy to use your somatic nervous system to pick up a pen. It's harder to slow your pounding heart before a presentation. Nevertheless, with practice, yoga, meditation, biofeedback and several other techniques (Chapter 5) allow you to influence your involuntary nervous system. Even taking a few deep breaths influences the autonomic nervous system: changes in the number of breaths you take can alter your heart rate by 12 to 15 beats per minute. As you breathe more deeply, more oxygen reaches your blood and your heart does not need to work as hard. The brain detects the increase in oxygen and autonomic nerves tell the heart that it doesn't need to pump as hard. This 'feedback' between mind and body means that it is hard to feel mentally stressed when your body is relaxed. So, you feel mentally calmer.

Biologists further divide the autonomic nervous system into 'sympathetic' and 'parasympathetic nerves', which have opposite actions. The balance between the activity of the sympathetic and parasympathetic nervous systems determines your arousal – and, therefore, your stress. When sympathetic activity dominates, arousal rises. When parasympathetic activity dominates, you feel more relaxed.

Sympathetic and parasympathetic nerves

Sympathetic activity increases when you are stressed or in danger. Sympathetic nerves increase the speed and force of your heartbeat, pumping more blood around your body. Your breathing becomes more rapid and deeper. Sympathetic nerves dilate the pupils, increase sweating and divert blood from the gut and skin to the muscles. Muscles surrounding the hair follicles tighten. That's why people turn pale and suffer goose bumps when they are frightened.

These changes are part of the 'fight-or-flight' response, which evolved to get us out of trouble quickly with the least possible damage. The fight-or-flight response was a lifesaver when a rival tribe on the warpath threatened our ancestors. Unfortunately, the response does not distinguish between barbarian hordes, a sabre-tooth cat, a pile of final demands or a nagging boss.

After a shock or when confronted with a threat, we enter the 'alarm' phase and the fight-or-flight response kicks in. The 'resistance' or adaptation phase follows and we take action to deal with the threat. If we succeed, the body returns to normal. However, our veneer of civilization prevents us from swinging a punch or fleeing the office. As a result, the flight-or-flight response remains active for long periods, depleting our emotional, physical and mental resources, and predisposing to mental and physical diseases.

In contrast, parasympathetic nerves slow the rate and reduce the force of the heart's contraction. The depth and speed of breathing declines. Blood flows back to the gut. In other words, rather than 'fight or take flight', parasympathetic nerves allow us to 'feed, breed and rest'.

Hormonal changes

Many organs release or respond to hormones and other chemical messengers to produce responses that are co-ordinated with the sympathetic and parasympathetic nervous systems. For example, sympathetic nerves stimulate your adrenal glands, which lie on top of your kidneys, to secrete hormones called adrenaline, noradrenaline and cortisol.

Adrenaline and noradrenaline (called epinephrine and norepinephrine in the USA) augment many elements in the fight-or-flight response, including raising heart and lung activity, slowing digestion and increasing levels of fat and glucose. Cortisol

The body's painkillers

The Sumerians, a civilization in southern Mesopotamia, used opium poppies to alleviate pain around 4000 BC. Some 6,000 years later, researchers in the 1970s discovered that the brain and some other parts of the body produce chemicals with the same painkilling, mood-lifting properties as opioids. Researchers call these natural opioids 'endorphins' (meaning 'morphine within') or 'enkephalins' (meaning 'in the head'). Endorphins explain why, remarkably, around 70 per cent of soldiers treated in front-line units for severe battle injuries and 40 per cent of people admitted after accidents to a city hospital did not report pain.[14]

also helps increase blood glucose levels (glucose is the fuel for your muscles and other organs). These hormonal changes seem to prolong the effects produced by the sympathetic nervous activity. Meanwhile, your brain produces painkillers to help you fight or run away even if you are injured.

The benefits of anxiety and depression

Anxiety and depression are the bane of many people's lives. Yet both probably evolved to help us adapt to danger. For example, the sense of anxiety, dread or panic heightens your vigilance – another manifestation of 'arousal' – if you are walking down a dark, lonely alley. The expectation of danger activates the fight-or-flight response preparing you to deal with a threat. Even depression may have benefits, including reducing your likelihood of engaging in risky behaviours.[15] Depression commonly follows pain – especially when chronic – and injury, and might reduce the chances of movement and, in turn, lower the risk of further damage. Anxiety and depression become 'diseases' when the severity, persistence or impact on your life becomes excessive.

Stress and the immune response

In the early twentieth century, the Russian scientist Ivan Pavlov rang a bell when he fed a dog. Faced with food, the dog salivated. Over time, the dog salivated when Pavlov rang the bell, whether or not he also offered food. Pavlov called this a 'conditioned reflex'.

Then, in the late 1970s, as Anne Harrington recounts in *The Cure Within*, scientists Robert Ader and Nicholas Cohen fed rats a mixture of water, saccharine and a drug called cyclophosphamide, which suppresses the immune system. When they stopped cyclophosphamide, but continued the water and saccharine mixture, the rats' immune responses remained impaired and they continued to die. In other words, the rats' impaired immune systems became 'conditioned' to the sweet taste of the saccharine.

Since then, scientists have uncovered numerous links between the nervous and immune systems. For example, lymphocytes – a type of white blood cell – produce small message-carrying proteins identical to some of those in the brain. As Harrington notes, this suggests the immune and nervous systems communicate. In addition, nerves hard-wire connections between the thymus gland, spleen, lymph nodes and bone marrow – all of which are important parts of the immune system. In 1980, Ader called the study of these connections 'psychoneuroimmunology'.

More than 30 years later, psychoneuroimmunology remains an area of active research helping us understand why stress can undermine the immune response. For example:

- Natural killer cells, another type of white blood cell, attack and destroy infected or cancerous cells. One study of students found that the activity of the natural killer cells declined around the time of their examinations.[16]
- Another study infected students experimentally with influenza virus. Stressed-out students suffered worse flu symptoms and produced more mucus than their less worried counterparts.[16]
- In carers looking after a husband or wife with dementia, levels of a cytokine (a type of biological messenger) that increases the activity of the immune system rose more quickly and persisted for longer after a flu vaccination than in less chronically stressed adults. Carers also generated lower levels of protective antibodies following a flu jab.[16]

This link between the nervous and immune systems produces a co-ordinated response that helps you recover from illness.

Spontaneous remission of cancer

The immune system destroys cancerous cells as well as invading bacteria, fungi and viruses. So, psychoneuroimmunology helps researchers understand a striking example of the intimate relationship between mind and body: spontaneous remissions of cancer.

Medically, spontaneous regression refers to the complete or partial disappearance of a malignancy when the patient is not receiving a treatment that could explain the improvement.[17] Some spontaneous remissions last for years. For example, spontaneous remissions in renal cell carcinoma – a malignancy in the kidney – have lasted between three months and 20 years. Nevertheless, most patients relapse[17] and regression rarely cures. On the other hand, metastatic cancer – a malignancy that has spread to other parts of the body – is generally incurable. Sadly, even the most effective modern treatment usually only buys you time.

Spontaneous remissions are more common than many patients and doctors realize and occur in almost every type of cancer.[17] Nevertheless, as Ventegodt and colleagues point out, many doctors seem unwilling to 'recognize, appreciate, and investigate' spontaneous remissions.[18] As a result, 'massive under-reporting' hinders attempts to work out how frequently spontaneous remissions occur. However, studies suggest that between one in every 100,000 and more than one in 10,000 cancers might spontaneously enter remission.[18] According to Cancer Research UK, doctors diagnosed 324,579 people with cancer during 2010. So, between 3 and 30 of these people potentially show spontaneous remission.

Interestingly, Ventegodt and colleagues remark that around two-thirds of patients experienced 'some kind of spiritual awakening' before the spontaneous remission – an issue we'll return to in the next chapter – suggesting that patients had 'a central role in the process of healing'.[18] Indeed, even if a cancer does not enter remission, a positive outlook seems to improve patients' prospects. In one study, women with early breast cancer who felt helpless, hopeless and depressed were 55 per cent more likely to die over the next five years than patients who managed to maintain a more positive outlook.[19] Numerous other examples illustrate the intimate link between the mind and body. One of these – the placebo effect – contributes to the benefit of every drug you take, every therapy you receive, every consultation about health you have, whether with a healthcare professional, a complementary healer or a counsellor.

The benevolent lie: the placebo enigma

A surgeon operating near the front line in the Korean War began to suffer severe pain in his abdomen. He knew he had developed acute appendicitis. However, incoming wounded needed his help. So, he asked the nurse to give him an injection of morphine. The pain eased and he kept working. With the crisis over, the doctor underwent surgery to remove the damaged appendix.[14]

After his return to duty, the doctor was looking through the operating room records and found that 'since he appeared distressed' the nurse had injected him with inactive saline and not morphine.[14] (She probably wanted to avoid the mental fogging that morphine can cause.) In other words, a simple salt solution used to mix injectable drugs alleviated the severe pain of acute appendicitis. Critically, however, the surgeon *expected* the nurse to follow his instructions and use the painkiller. And this expectation invoked the placebo effect.

The term 'placebo' derives from the Latin phrase 'I shall please'. For important funerals, medieval people sometimes hired mourners, who often recited a verse from Psalm 114: *placebo Domino in regione vivorum* – or 'I shall please the Lord in the land of the living'. As professional mourners often replaced the deceased's family members, 'placebo' began to carry a connotation of substitution. By 1811, 'placebo' had come to mean 'any medicine adapted more to please than benefit the patient'.[20]

Placebos soon became a mainstay of medicine – especially as contemporary drugs were often ineffective, but could still cause side effects. In the early years of the twentieth century, doctors used a variety of multi-coloured sugar pills, bread pills and water injected into the fat beneath the skin as placebos – especially if the doctor regarded the patient as 'unintelligent, neurotic or inadequate'.[20] In the 1950s, the *British Medical Journal* reported that 40 per cent of patients in general practice received placebos.[21]

Today, we know that the placebo response contributes to the effectiveness and side effects of every drug you take, every complementary treatment you try, every lifestyle change you make. For example:

- In a study of 55 patients with mild asthma, a placebo bronchodilator (a drug that opens asthmatic airways) reduced the lungs' reactivity to asthma triggers. The placebo improved asthmatic symptoms in 18 per cent of patients.[22]
- Irritable bowel syndrome (IBS) causes stomach cramps and pain, bloating, diarrhoea and constipation. On average, placebo responses account for around 40 per cent of the benefit of an IBS treatment. However, depending on the study, the placebo response can vary between 16 per cent and 71 per cent.[23]
- An analysis that included 75 studies of antidepressants found that up to half of people taking placebo improved markedly. Furthermore, between a quarter and a third of people with agoraphobia or panic disorder responded to placebo.[21]

- Two hours after taking soluble aspirin, 27 per cent of migraine sufferers were pain-free, compared to 33 per cent with ibuprofen and 37 per cent with sumatriptan (a drug for migraine). The placebo response rate was 13 per cent.[24]
- Sleep latency (the time taken to fall asleep) declined by 42 minutes in patients taking eszopiclone, zaleplon or zolpidem for insomnia. The placebo effect accounted for approximately half this reduction.[25]

As a result, well-designed studies of medicines include a placebo – an inert drug that looks identical but does not contain any active ingredient.

Placebo responses also contribute to the effectiveness of complementary medicine. In one study, 71 per cent of migraines responded entirely or partially during the two hours after inhaling lavender essential oil. However, 47 per cent improved with placebo.[26] In another study, 32 per cent of people taking a mixture of feverfew (a herb traditionally used to alleviate headaches) and ginger (traditionally used to counter nausea, common in people with migraines) for migraine were pain-free two hours after treatment compared to 16 per cent for placebo.[27] Lavender oil and the combination of feverfew and ginger were more effective than placebo. Yet the placebo accounts for about half the benefit. So why are placebos so effective?

Mummy will kiss it better

The promise that 'Mummy will kiss it better' is, effectively, a placebo. Most children trust their mothers: they expect their parents to make things better. And so the symptoms abate. As we get older, we expect our doctors to help. So, those doctors who raise our expectations and invoke our optimism, who are enthusiastic about the treatment, who are confident, authoritative, empathic, charismatic and warm seem to bolster the placebo effect and enhance the treatment's intrinsic activity.[21, 14]

On the other side of the relationship, a patient's desire to believe, 'obey' and please the doctor tends to enhance the placebo response.[21] Not surprisingly, hostility reduces a drug's efficacy,[14] partly by countering the placebo benefit and partly by making poor adherence (page 15) more likely.

Similarly, patients expect high-tech, expensive medical equipment to produce marked biological benefits. By the late 1980s, several studies had suggested that ultrasound reduced pain, jaw swelling and tightness after the extraction of wisdom teeth. So one study varied the intensity of ultrasound, but did not tell either the therapist or the patient what 'dose' the machine delivered. Patients benefited even when the machine did not produce any ultrasound. Indeed, the benefits when the machine was switched off were often more marked than when the machine produced the usual intensity of ultrasound.[14]

At first, researchers speculated that the massage of the jaw with the head of the ultrasound machine might account for the benefits. However, training patients to massage themselves with the inactive ultrasound head using the same movements as the therapists did not alleviate the pain and swelling. As Wall points out, the benefit 'required an impressive machine and someone in a white coat to transmit the effect'.[14]

Pill colour, football and placebos

Even the shape and the colour of a drug can influence the placebo effect. For example, most people regard blue tablets as a depressant – after all, we get the 'blues'.[21] Placebo capsules containing coloured beads reduce pain more effectively than coloured placebo tablets.[14] And coloured placebo tablets are more effective than white tablets with corners. In turn, white tablets with corners are more effective than round white tablets.[14]

A network of mutually reinforcing factors seems to account for these benefits. For example, most people regard red or orange tablets as stimulant[21] – perhaps because the colours are associated with danger. An 'inactive' injection of saline is more effective than a placebo tablet of any colour.[14] We expect an injection to deliver a more potent drug. Indeed, one doctor boosted the power of his placebo by handling the tablets with forceps, telling the patient that the medicine was too powerful to touch.[14]

Culture and society also influence the power of a placebo. Patients expect modern medicine to be effective – especially when supported by the power of advertising. Placebos taken from a bottle labelled with a well-known brand are more effective painkillers than those from a bottle with a typed label.[14] Similarly, a study from Italy showed that blue tablets were sedatives in women, but caused insomnia among men. The researchers suggested that, in general, women might associate blue with the comfort of the Virgin Mary. Many men, on the other hand, associate the colour with the excitement of the Italian national soccer team.[21] In other words, the power of placebo depends on patients' 'culture, background, experience and personality'.[14]

Not all in the mind

But culture, background, experience and personality don't fully account for placebo's benefits: placebos also produce a range of demonstrable biological changes. For example, placebo analgesics can counter pain by increasing endogenous opioid levels (page 24)[14] and dampening inflammation. Placebos also counter anxiety and depression,[21] which exacerbate any given level of discomfort.

On the other hand, going to a doctor and receiving a treatment relieves anxiety (partly by validating the 'sick role'; see page 20), while placebos evoke positive, optimistic thoughts, which help counter depression.[21] As a result, placebos can reduce the emotional aspects of pain without affecting the sensation itself.[21] This reassurance also reduces the activity of the sympathetic nervous system, reflected in a decline in blood pressure. In one study, a drug called nebivolol reduced blood pressure by between 7.8 mmHg and 9.1 mmHg, depending on the dose. Placebo reduced blood pressure by 4.6 mmHg. In other words, the placebo accounted for about half the drug's effect.[28]

In addition, Russell notes that up to 90 per cent of acute (short-lived) diseases improve regardless of the treatment (in other words, they are self-limiting). Asthma attacks can wax and wane as exposure to the trigger varies. A flare of pain and inflammation in an arthritic joint can abate. A headache passes. Over time, the flares and remissions average out. Doctors call this the 'regression to the mean' (mean is another word for average). Again, this contributes to the placebo effect: you tend to ascribe the change to the treatment rather than the body's innate healing abilities.

Curses and the nocebo effect

Unfortunately, the placebo effect can prove a double-edged sword. In the middle of the nineteenth century, a Maori woman accidentally ate fruit harvested from a place covered by a taboo (*tapu*). When, in the afternoon, she learnt that she had broken the *tapu*, she claimed that the chief's spirit would kill her. Sure enough, she was dead by noon the following day. In an influential article published in 1942, Walter Cannon from Harvard Medical School noted that the Maori *tapu* is potentially so potent that even a strong young man could die the same day as he broke the taboo. Cannon describes the *tapu* as 'a fatal power of the imagination working through unmitigated terror'.[29]

Numerous other examples from around the world suggest that if the person believes strongly enough in the power of magic, curses can induce disease and even death. For example, in Australian Aboriginal cultures, a curse can leave the victim living in terror – which psychiatrist Harry Eastwell, who reported his experiences of treating 39 victims, called 'sorcery-induced fear'. Indeed, people who believe that they are cursed often exhibit many hallmarks of increased sympathetic nervous system activity (page 23), such as intense agitation, marked restlessness, heavy sweating, heightened vigilance, and so on. In three of the 39 patients Eastwell treated, the fear was so intense that their eyeballs protruded, with widely dilated pupils.[30]

It's a long way from traditional Maori or Aboriginal societies to the medicines you take. Yet just as the Aboriginal people believe that curses cause harm, we believe that medicines cause side effects, which can become a self-fulfilling prophecy. Indeed, doctors increasingly discuss possible side effects to help patients make informed decisions about treatment. Yet informing a patient that a drug might cause a side effect may produce the same adverse event independently of the medicine's action.[31]

Doctors call this effect the 'nocebo' – from the Latin for 'I shall harm'. For example, a group of medicines for depression called tri-cyclic antidepressants (TCA) are more likely to cause certain adverse events than another class called selective serotonin reuptake inhibitors (SSRIs). People who received TCA placebos were around three times more likely to report dry mouth, drowsiness and constipation, and about twice as likely to report sexual problems (all side effects linked to TCAs) than those using SSRI placebos.[32] Similarly, between 4 and 26 per cent of patients taking placebos for statins – a group of drugs used to lower raised levels of cholesterol – stopped taking their treatment as they thought they had developed adverse events.[31]

As this chapter shows, overwhelming scientific evidence shows that the mind influences the body and vice versa – the principle underpinning holistic health. Even if stress does not cause a disease, feeling anxious, worried and wound up can certainly make you feel worse. The message is clear: keeping a positive attitude and staying relaxed helps bolster your inner healer.

3

The spirit in medicine

As we have seen, scientific biomedicine is responsible for many health advances we take for granted, from vaccinations to anti-biotics to life-saving care after a heart attack. But despite its success, scientific medicine does not fully encompass the plethora of 'psy-chological, sociological, and spiritual factors' that contribute to 'most, if not all, illnesses'.[1] Science is unsurpassed at identifying targets for new treatments for a range of malignancies; it is less effective at helping you rebuild your life after you receive the dev-astating news that you have cancer.

To get your life back on track, you'll need a holistic approach encompassing a healthy lifestyle (Chapter 4), resilience (Chapter 7) and spirituality. As theologian Philip Sheldrake notes, spir-ituality broadens how we understand and experience healing and disease. (Sheldrake's *Spirituality: A very short introduction* is a brilliant place to start exploring this complex area.) For instance, spirituality helps people use suffering, even if incur-able, as a means to growth. 'Spiritual health care' also places greater emphasis than conventional medicine on the connections between the person and the environment and, Sheldrake says, understands illness as having 'complex causes, including personal and social contexts' – which is the theme that underlies this book.

The continuing importance of religion

Spirituality is part of being human. More than 40,000 years ago, Neanderthal and Palaeolithic man engaged in complex religious rituals, seemed to suggest they understood the idea of death and drew images of mythical creatures on cave walls.[2] As Polkinghorne points out: 'At almost all times and in almost all places, human beings have participated in an admittedly bafflingly diverse history of encounters with the sacred.'

Some researchers believe that the need for spirituality is hard-wired into the human brain.[2, 3] Genes seem to account for about half of the differences between people in their religiousness, spiritual feelings and beliefs. (The genes could contain the instructions for building the 'spirituality pathways' in the brain, for example.) That's about the same as the genetic impact on intelligence. This suggests that, from an evolutionary perspective, religious experiences must increase the chances of survival.[2] Certainly, as we'll see later in the chapter, religion seems to increase the likelihood of a long and healthy life.

This hard-wiring and genetic predisposition may help explain why, despite the supposed rise of secularism and atheism, only about a quarter of the population in England and Wales did not state a religion in the 2011 census. However, identifying yourself with a religion is not necessarily the same as being religious or spiritual. Some people are lapsed or non-practising. Others regard themselves as 'Christians', for example, but attend church only for baptisms, weddings and funerals – and, at a push, Easter and Christmas.

British religious diversity

Overall, 59 per cent of people in England and Wales regard themselves as Christian, almost 5 per cent as Muslim and 1.5 per cent as Hindu, according to the 2011 census. In addition, 0.8 per cent – about one in every 125 – are Sikh, 0.5 per cent Jewish and 0.4 per cent Buddhist. But the proportions vary across the country. In the North East of England, 68 per cent of people regard themselves as Christian, while 12 per cent of the population in London are Muslim and 2 per cent of people in the West Midlands are Sikh.

In other words, religion and spirituality (we will look at the difference in the next section) help many people find meaning in their lives. A survey of 7,403 people in England found that 35 per cent understood life through religion and 19 per cent were spiritual but not religious. Less than half (46 per cent) were neither religious nor spiritual.[4] And growing scientific evidence suggests that religious activities and integrating spirituality more closely into your everyday activities can improve the quality, and even the quantity, of your life, without entering a monastery, attending church every day or passing hours in meditation.

Religion versus spirituality

Religion and spirituality overlap – but are not identical. Some people, such as those who see religion as a 'social' obligation, attend religious services regularly but are decidedly unspiritual. On the other hand, some deeply spiritual people do not follow a 'recognized' religion.

Differentiating religion and spirituality taxes theologians. But essentially, religion refers to a group's collective spiritual experiences based around organized beliefs and practices. The word 'religion' derives from the Latin word *religare*, 'to bind together'.[1]

Spirituality – from the Latin *spiritualitas*, meaning 'breath' – covers a much wider range of beliefs, experiences and values than any one religion. Sheldrake comments that, broadly, spirituality refers to 'lifestyles and practices that embody a vision of human existence and of how the human spirit is to achieve its full potential'. He adds that spirituality is 'holistic . . . a fully integrated approach to life'. The National Cancer Institute defines spirituality as 'an individual's sense of peace, purpose, and connection to others, and beliefs about the meaning of life'. So, spirituality refers to personal practices and attitudes that typically:

- foster and promote 'connections' with yourself and others;
- include a search for life's meaning and purpose;
- offer a cohesive system of values, usually encompassing love (in the broadest sense), compassion and justice.

In other words, spirituality is a personal search, alone or in a group. The search can follow a single path – as with an organized religion. However, some people 'pick' from a spiritual smorgasbord, choosing elements from various traditions. This diversity means that everyone can probably find a set of spiritual values that 'works for them'. However, followers of conventional religions often criticize this 'pick and mix approach' to spirituality. And this variety makes studying spirituality's effect on mental and physical health notoriously difficult. A pagan worshipping the Earth mother, a Zen Buddhist and a Sikh may all be deeply spiritual. But isolating the influence of their lifestyles, personality and psychology from the impact of their spirituality is almost impossible.

To try to reduce the confusion, many investigations study the health benefits associated with organized religions, which have a consistent core of beliefs. However, the benefits of religions extend beyond the spiritual. For example, they offer a sense of community and friendship (Chapter 6), practical support and a structured lifestyle (such as health-promoting dietary restrictions or bans on drugs and alcohol) that might help account for at least some of their benefits on health and well-being.

Furthermore, religions may bolster the benefits of conventional medicine. Some religions engender a 'respect' for authority, which increases the chances that people will follow their doctor's advice. Indeed, people who report higher levels of spiritual well-being are more likely to take their medicine as their doctors suggest.[5] Religious leaders can also reassure people that the treatment offered does not conflict with the religious texts and reinforce health promotion messages.

Spirituality and holistic health

Such complications notwithstanding, spirituality and religion undoubtedly improve holistic health. One analysis included 42 studies that examined the relationship between religious involvement and deaths from any cause. Being deeply religious and regularly involved in religion reduced the risk of death by 29 per cent.[6] Indeed, religion and spirituality seem to protect against a range of diseases:

- Secular Jewish men were around four times more likely to suffer their first heart attack than Orthodox Jews, even allowing for other risk factors such as age, smoking, body mass index (BMI – see page 71) and physical activity. The link was even more marked – around a seven-fold increase – among women.[1]
- Orthodox Jewish men were 20 per cent less likely to die from coronary heart disease than nonreligious men, again after allowing for risk factors such as age, blood pressure, levels of fat in the blood, smoking, diabetes and BMI.
- People who prayed or participated in other private religious activities were 40 per cent less likely to have hypertension than

those who attended religious services infrequently or who did not engage in private religious activities.[1]

- Spirituality improved psychological well-being, quality of life and self-rated health among patients with kidney disease undergoing dialysis.[7]
- As mentioned previously (page 27), around two-thirds of patients experienced 'some kind of spiritual awakening' before the spontaneous remission of cancer.[8]
- Patients who report paranormal experiences and beliefs tend to be healthier than those with more mainstream views. Paranormal experiences and beliefs – which are often allied to spirituality – can help some people understand life crises and bolster mental health.[9]

The link between spirituality and health

Various factors probably contribute to the link between spirituality and religion and holistic health. For example, among people with cancer, higher levels of spiritual well-being enhanced hope and their ability to cope and function socially. Limiting the impact of cancer on daily life seems to prolong survival (pages 27 and 102). Indeed, more spiritual people also rated their health and quality of life as being better than their less spiritual counterparts, which helps explain why the cancer seemed to trigger less psychological stress, depression, financial strain and suicidal thoughts.[5]

This ability to bolster our defences against stress is probably one reason why religious people are less likely to become addicted to drink and drugs than their more secular counterparts. In an English study, religious people were 27 per cent less likely to have ever used drugs and 19 per cent less likely to put their health at risk by drinking heavily than those who were neither religious nor spiritual.[4]

Religion and spirituality also help people cast off the shackles of addiction. For example, former problem drinkers who integrated religious and spiritual activities into their daily life were more likely to remain sober than those who did not, even after allowing for participation in Alcoholics Anonymous. Private religious and spiritual practices (such as prayer and reading spiritual texts) and forgiving themselves (most drinkers suffer profound guilt about the harm they have done to themselves and others) were especially effective. In fact, including spirituality in former drinkers' daily lives predicted their chance of long-term sobriety more strongly than their levels of stress or contentment.[10] Indeed, Sheldrake comments, drug and alcohol services increasingly treat addictions as spiritual diseases. He adds that the 12-step programme used by, among others, Alcoholics Anonymous 'encourage[s] a personal belief system based on spiritual self-discovery'.

For many people, drink or drug abuse is a sign of a general, profound dissatisfaction or helps them 'cope' with emotional or mental problems. When they stop drinking the void remains – and, in many cases, the addiction has deepened the emotional and psychological chasm. So they switch to another addiction to fill the gap, such as overeating, compulsive shopping or excessive exercise. However, religious and spiritual practices help fill the void and reduce the risk that they'll swap one addiction for another.

In addition, many people who drink excessively or abuse drugs are emotionally vulnerable and have chaotic lives. In some cases, the devastation wrought by drink and drugs leaves them emotionally and mentally vulnerable. However, many people drink excessively or use drugs *because* they are emotionally and mentally vulnerable.

This void, their recognition of their vulnerability and problems finding meaning in their suffering means that some people seek solace in New Age beliefs or change religions. Everyone has to find their own spiritual path. However, because they are especially vulnerable and need practical advice and support, people recovering from addictions or trying to live with a mental illness may benefit more from organized religion than a more unstructured spirituality.

For example, an English study found that spiritual people were 77 per cent more likely to be dependent on drugs than those who were neither religious nor spiritual. Spiritual people were also more likely to have abnormal eating attitudes (by 46 per cent), generalized anxiety disorder (50 per cent) or a phobia (72 per cent). Spiritual people were also 40 per cent more likely to be taking a medicine for a psychiatric illness.[4]

It seems unlikely – outside cults or using psychotropic drugs to 'open the doors of perception' – that spiritual practices cause the drink and drug abuse. If you're well-adjusted, exploring the spiritual smorgasbord can be exciting, stimulating and inspiring, and, as Sheldrake notes, spiritualities that are detached from traditions and established beliefs appeal to some people. However, he argues that these 'tend to bypass issues of commitment' and may not help people examine human meaning in the same way as the insights offered by long-standing religions, which have 'highly developed' spiritual traditions. As such, some people with alcohol, drug and other mental problems might be better in a more organized framework offering security, structure and support. And many religiously based charities offer invaluable experience gained helping thousands of people. Overcoming addiction is tough and addicts need all the help they can get.

Towards the end of life

As the long tradition of deathbed conversions shows, many people find that religion and spirituality become increasingly important towards the end of life. Indeed, John Vayalilkarottu, from the

The stages of dying

Psychiatrist Elisabeth Kübler-Ross developed a now widely accepted view of grief or catastrophic personal loss (such as divorce, unemployment and imprisonment) that suggests people typically pass through five emotional stages:

- Denial and isolation – a common initial response to receiving bad news.
- Anger – patients ask, 'Why me?' Carers often bear the brunt of this anger.
- Bargaining – patients try to postpone or delay the event, perhaps by prayer or a secret pact with God.
- Depression – this can emerge as a 'reaction' to the grief and loss as well as a reaction to treatment and physical problems.
- Acceptance – the patient reaches peace. Some patients and their caregivers are even able to find 'meaning' in their illness and use the disease as impetus towards spiritual growth (page 100).

The order varies from person to person. You may experience more than one stage at a time. And you may move to and fro between stages.

Australian Catholic University, notes, 'In the face of daunting fear; famine, sickness, disaster or death, religion has always been a wellspring of hope.'[3] For example, a study of cancer patients receiving radiotherapy to alleviate symptoms rather than cure the malignancy (palliation) found that 84 per cent used religious or spiritual beliefs to help them cope.[11] People who participate in religious activities at the end of their lives tend to accept their death more readily than the less religiously inclined, irrespective of their belief in an afterlife.[1]

Against this background, the World Health Organization stresses that palliative medicine should encompass psychosocial and spiritual care as well as management of physical symptoms.[1] Indeed, in some cases, spiritual beliefs may influence the choice of treatment for pain and other physical symptoms. (Some people want to go gently into that good night fully aware. Opiates can cause mental cloudiness.) Because the end of life is deeply personal, doctors and nurses individualize palliative care.

So, let your family and doctors know your spiritual and religious preferences – even if that means 'admitting' that the spiritual 'crisis' evoked by a fatal illness has overturned life-long beliefs. How would you like your body to be treated after death? What funeral arrangements would you like? Would you want to receive powerful painkillers at the point of death? You could try talking to your spiritual leader, specialist or hospice, or a support group such as Macmillan Cancer Support. Even if you have not attended religious services regularly or had contact with spiritual leaders, both can be an invaluable source of emotional and practical support for you and your loved ones. If a loved one is dying, gently ask for his or her preferences. If you find this difficult, you could see if a doctor or counsellor could help.

Helping those left behind

Not surprisingly, the death of a loved one can prove especially difficult practically, psychologically, spiritually and emotionally. In some cases, you'll obviously miss a loved one. However, grief can be profound even if the relationship was difficult during life: you may grieve for the relationship you never had and now never can have.

During terminal illness, you might want to make the most of the time left. However, you might find that your loved one becomes withdrawn. In some cases, depression may trigger the withdrawal, in which case the doctor or nurse may be able to help. In other cases, losing interest in things and people around you, even close family, is a natural part of gradually withdrawing from the world. So, your 'needs' at this difficult time can differ from those of the terminally ill person.

You will need to find your own way through this tough period in your life. You could look back and see how you managed with previous stressful experiences. What helped you cope when, for example, a parent, grandparent or close friend died? What proved a problem? (This helps you develop proactive strategies to tackle the practical problems.) Did you cope by drinking excessively? What will you tell your children?

Drawing on a religious leader's advice, experience and support can bolster your mental, physical and emotional health. One study interviewed people caring for a loved one with advanced cancer. All caregivers considered themselves spiritual and 98 per cent considered themselves religious. All said that spirituality and religiosity helped them cope; 58 per cent said that spirituality and religiosity alleviated their loved one's physical symptoms and 76 per cent said that spirituality and religiosity helped the emotional symptoms.[12]

Nonetheless, 58 per cent of caregivers reported spiritual pain, which meant they were unable to find meaning, hope, love, peace, comfort, strength and so on in their religion, or said that conflict arose between their beliefs and experiences. Understandably, spiritual pain increased the risk that the caregiver would suffer anxiety, depression or denial, or would use other dysfunctional coping strategies (page 104) and undermined caregivers' quality of life.[12] Caregivers need to care for themselves (page 93).

Finally, give yourself permission to grieve and don't expect life to get 'back to normal' too quickly. Profound sadness, a deep sense of loss, sleeplessness, crying, inability to concentrate, tiredness and poor appetite are part of normal grief. They don't mean that you're mentally ill. In other words, don't be afraid to cry: tears discharge tension generated by sadness. According to one estimate, 'resolving' the loss of a loved pet means crying for at least 20 hours. 'Resolving' (you never overcome) the loss of a spouse, parent, child or close friend requires 200–300 hours of crying.[13] Occasionally, however, grief goes beyond the 'normal' response to bereavement.

You may, for example, develop depression, abuse drugs or alcohol, feel 'dead' or 'unreal', find you can't work or take part in your normal activities several weeks after the death, or suffer symptoms of post-traumatic stress disorder (page 100). If you think your grief is abnormal, speak to your GP or a counsellor: medicines or psychological interventions, such as guided mourning, often help.

Talking to your spiritual leader, a counsellor or a member of the palliative care team can also help you cope emotionally and practically with a death. Bereavement means dealing with numerous practical issues as you rebuild your life, including wills, money and benefits. Cruse or the Child Bereavement Trust offer specific counselling for bereaved people.

Side effects of religion and spirituality

In common with any approach to bolstering holistic health, a deep involvement in religion can have unintended consequences. For example, some religious beliefs may mean people avoid or stop conventional health care.[1] Jehovah's Witnesses might not accept a blood transfusion. People from some cultures may resort to traditional healers (medicine and religion are often intertwined). Indeed, spiritual people from the industrialized world may prefer alternative medicines and stop their conventional treatments. Religious and cultural beliefs – as well as modesty and embarrassment – stop some women from undergoing breast or cervical cancer screening.

In addition, some religious people may hold unrealistically high expectations for themselves and others, which can lead to isolation, stress and anxiety. In other cases, members of a religious community may isolate themselves from other people who do not share their beliefs.[1] And some people may feel that the illness is God's punishment for a perceived sin, which may make it more difficult to adapt to serious illness.

Indeed, you can have too much faith: God helps those who help themselves. An American study found that people who used religious coping strategies following a heart attack were more likely to experience depression while in hospital and over the following month. Some people seem to 'over-rely' on their relationship with God to aid their recovery, which can develop into a form of fatalism. Recovering from a heart attack depends on taking a more active approach to care – accepting medical treatments and following medical instructions – than is the case with many chronic diseases.[14]

Nevertheless, religion and spirituality are essential elements in holistic health.

The prayer conundrum

According to Polkinghorne, the healing of the sick is 'the most characteristic action attributed to Jesus in the course of his public ministry'. Polkinghorne notes that at least some of the healing miracles reflect the 'influence of an exceptionally gifted charismatic healer'. However, an especially marked placebo effect (page 27) doesn't explain all the stories, particularly healing at a distance, an issue considered later in the chapter. And 2,000 years later, millions of people still pray for a 'healing miracle' – and St Peregrine, the Lourdes pilgrims and millions of others worldwide believe that God sometimes answers.

In some ways, the link isn't that surprising. After all, praying for someone shows you care. Praying, or knowing someone cares enough to pray for you, may make you feel better by enhancing well-being, optimism and confidence[15] and bolstering the body's innate ability to heal itself.

For example, proximal intercessory prayer (PIP) involves touch – such as placing hands on the patient's head or embracing him or her – and praying close to that person. Often those leading the prayers are confident, authoritative, empathic and charismatic, which, as we've seen (page 27), bolsters the placebo effect.[16, 17] In one study, PIP by evangelical Christians improved auditory and visual acuity in patients from rural Mozambique with poor hearing and sight. PIP's effects were greater than those produced by suggestion or hypnosis, which can sharpen auditory and visual acuity.[18]

The 'problem' of intercessory prayer

More controversially, at least for scientists, several studies suggest that intercessory prayer at a distance speeds healing. In 1988, doctors in San Francisco split 393 patients admitted to a coronary care unit into two groups. The first group received no organized prayer, while Christians outside the hospital prayed for the second group's recovery. When admitted, the two groups were equally ill. But the intercessory prayer group developed less severe heart disease, were less likely to need mechanical help breathing, and consumed fewer antibiotics and diuretics (water tablets).[19] In 1999, researchers in Kansas City found that distant intercessory prayer reduced the severity of heart disease by 11 per cent.[20]

Other studies tell a similar story. In a study of 26 people left *unconscious* (so they had no idea they were being prayed for) after severe head injuries, patients recovered better if they were the subject of intercessory prayer.[21] Another investigation examined bush babies (a small African primate) that had injured themselves (as in humans, a sign of distress). Self-inflicted wounds healed quicker in bush babies who were intercessory prayer subjects compared to animals who were not. The intercessory prayer group also showed improved blood quality – such as increased red blood cells and haemoglobin (the chemical in the blood that carries oxygen around the body) – and more time spent in normal behaviours, such as grooming.[22] Obviously, bush babies do not have the strongly held beliefs about religion and medicine that influence the placebo effect.

Furthermore, some studies suggest that other distance healing techniques – including spiritual healing, noncontact therapeutic touch and external qi gong (page 78) – also seem to work. For example, in AIDS patients, distance healing reduced the likelihood of new AIDS-related illnesses (by 83 per cent), visits to doctors (by 30 per cent), hospitalizations (by 75 per cent) and time spent in hospital (by 85 per cent).[23] In 2000, researchers examined 23 trials involving 2,774 patients. Thirteen studies suggested that various types of distance healing worked.[24]

Many religious and spiritual people will take these results as confirming that their beliefs are right. Cynics and atheists suggest that there is something 'wrong' with the studies, that they were biased in some way, that the method was flawed, or both. You are free to draw your own conclusions about distance healing and intercessory prayer. However, there is no doubt that bolstering your spiritual side is one of the most effective ways to enhance your holistic health and improve your quality – and perhaps quantity – of life.

4

Four steps to help your inner healer

Fundamentally, holistic health means tackling the plethora of physical, emotional, spiritual and environmental factors that undermine your health and well-being. As complementary healers often point out, there is no point in expecting, for example, acupuncture to help a cough if you continue to smoke. Or, as the sixteenth-century proverb remarks, 'God helps those that help themselves.'

So, in addition to taking your medicine, you need to look at your lifestyle. If you have a chronic disease, you and your healthcare team will work together to devise lifestyle changes tailored for you. (The recommendations in this chapter are suggestions. If you have a chronic illness, you should always confirm the change with your doctor.)

Four elements form the foundation of a healthy lifestyle: adequate exercise; quitting smoking; avoiding excessive alcohol consumption; and a healthy diet. We will not look at these in detail – plenty of other books show you how to build these strong foundations. But this chapter outlines the most important principles that can boost your holistic health.

Why you need to take a holistic approach

The landmark INTERHEART study underscored the importance of taking a holistic approach to a healthy lifestyle. INTERHEART compared the lifestyles of 15,152 patients from 52 countries who had suffered their first heart attack and 14,820 people who had never experienced a heart attack. Nine factors accounted for 90 per cent of the risk of the first heart attack among men and 94 per cent among women (see Table 4.1).[1]

INTERHEART showed that many heart attack risk factors 'cluster', which underscores the importance of a holistic approach. For example, many people comfort eat high-fat and sugary foods when they feel anxious or depressed. So, they are more likely to be over-

Table 4.1 Risk and protective factors against first heart attack in INTERHEART

Risk factors	Hypertension
	Diabetes
	Smoking
	Dangerous profile of cholesterol and other fats in blood
	Psychosocial factors (such as stress and depression)
	Abdominal obesity ('a bulging waistline')
Protective factors	Eating fruits and vegetables daily
	Regular exercise
	Regular (moderate) alcohol consumption

weight or obese. In turn, overweight or obese people are more likely to develop a range of diseases including diabetes, hypertension and depression. And depression increases the likelihood of comfort eating, avoiding exercise and so gaining weight.[2] Similarly, some people smoke to counter stress.

INTERHEART found that the more of these risk factors you have, the greater your likelihood of suffering a heart attack. Compared to people without any of the nine risk factors:

- people with diabetes who smoke and have hypertension are 13 times more likely to suffer a heart attack;
- those with five risk factors (harmful levels of cholesterol and other fats, obesity, smoking, diabetes and hypertension) are almost 69 times more likely to have a heart attack;
- people who suffer psychosocial problems in addition to the other five risk factors are about 334 times more likely to suffer a heart attack.[1]

Stress and heart disease

INTERHEART also found that psychosocial factors (such as stress and depression) roughly trebled the risk of having a heart attack.[1] INTERHEART defined stress as feeling irritable, being filled with anxiety or having difficulty sleeping because of problems. The researchers looked at stress over the year before the study and separated, as far as possible:

- stress at work
- stress at home
- stress caused by financial problems
- major stressful life events (such as divorce, business failure, unemployment or death of a spouse).

After allowing for other risk factors (e.g. age, sex and smoking), they found that:

- patients who experienced several periods of work-related stress were 38 per cent more likely to suffer a heart attack;
- experiencing several periods of stress at home increased the risk by 52 per cent;
- heart attack risk roughly doubled among those who endured permanent stress at work or home;
- severe financial stress increased the likelihood of a heart attack by 33 per cent (page 17);
- stressful life events increased heart attack risk by 48 per cent;
- feeling depressed for at least two weeks in the year before the study increased heart attack risk by 55 per cent.[3]

Strong emotions and heart health

Other studies confirm that psychological factors can profoundly undermine our heart's health. For example, negative and positive emotions increased the risk of a heart attack 4.5 and 3.5 times respectively over the following 2 to 24 hours.[4] An analysis of six studies found that high levels of perceived stress increased the risk of being diagnosed with, hospitalization for or dying from coronary heart disease by 27 per cent, which is broadly equivalent to smoking five more cigarettes per day.[5]

Once again, the relationship between mind and body runs both ways. For example, depressed patients are almost seven times more likely to die from heart disease or suffer a non-fatal heart attack during the next year than those who were not depressed.[6] Furthermore, depression increased the risk of death over the six months after a heart attack around four-fold.[7]

Although these examples focus on heart attacks, factors interact to increase the risk of many other diseases. That's why a lifestyle that bolsters holistic health can reduce the risk of developing serious illness and augment the benefits of conventional and complementary treatments for chronic diseases.

Exercise

Exercise increases mobility, strength and stamina, and helps protect against osteoporosis, hypertension, heart attacks, strokes and so on. Exercise also helps you maintain your ideal weight. You should be moderately active for at least 30 minutes on at least five days – and ideally every day – a week. It does not all have to be in one go. You can exercise for 15 minutes twice a day, for example.

You should aim to exercise until you are breathing harder than usual, but not so hard that you can't hold a conversation. You should feel that your heart is beating faster than usual and you have begun to sweat. However, if you experience chest pain or feel faint or otherwise unwell, stop exercising and see your doctor.

Exercise as part of everyday life

You should aim to make exercise part of your everyday life. If you exercise regularly for a year, you will lose about half your cardio-vascular fitness in just three months if you stop. So, find a type of exercise that you enjoy and that fits into your lifestyle – and stick with it. If you do not like exercise classes and you join a gym some distance from home or work, you are more likely to quit. On the other hand, you can easily integrate walking into your daily life. A pedometer helps ensure you walk at least 10,000 steps a day, as recommended by the American Heart Association.

There are plenty of other opportunities make exercise part of your day-to-day life:

- Walk to the local shops instead of taking the car.
- Ride a bike to work instead of travelling by car or public transport.
- Park a 15-minute walk from your place of work.
- If you take the bus, tube or metro, get off one or two stops early.
- Use the stairs instead of the lift.
- Clean the house regularly and wash your car by hand.
- Grow your own vegetables – and they taste better.
- Buy a pet. Apart from their other holistic health benefits (Chapter 6) walking the dog, riding and so on encourage exercise.

Back to nature

You should also try to get out of town. Strolling around country parks and nature reserves brings other benefits besides just boosting fitness. As Sheldrake points out, intense experiences evoked by, for example, music, nature and even some sciences (such as astrophysics, cosmology and, I'd argue, evolutionary biology) can create 'self-transcendent wonder' that's akin to spirituality.

As mentioned in the introduction, patients who had a view of a natural setting recovered from surgery more rapidly than a similar group who faced a wall.[8] Similarly, Japanese people with chronic illness often benefit from walking in woods – called *shinrin-yoku* (forest bathing). Scientific studies suggest that, among other benefits, *shinrin-yoku* encourages relaxation, reduces stress, lowers blood pressure and boosts the immune system. Even looking at, for example, a picture of people walking in a forest reduced blood pressure. But the smell and other sensations of walking through a forest augment the visual appreciation of natural beauty.[9]

So, make the most of the more than 400 country parks and many other nature reserves in England alone. The following are good places to start:

- Natural England: <www.naturalengland.org.uk/ourwork/ enjoying/places/countryparks/countryparksnetwork/ findacountrypark>
- The National Trust:
- The Ramblers: <www.ramblers.org.uk/go-walking.aspx>
- The Royal Society for the Protection of Birds: <www.rspb.org.uk/ reserves>
- The Woodland Trust: <visitwoods.org.uk>.

Smoking and drinking

Unless you have struggled with being hooked on a legal or illegal drug, it's easy to dismiss addiction, dependency and heavy use as lifestyle choices. But addiction erodes the person's ability to say no. The compulsion overwhelms good intentions and lays siege to every intellectual, rational and emotional defence the user can muster, until he or she can no longer resist addiction's assault.

Addiction offers a striking example of the intimate link between mind, body and environment. For example, abnormalities in the part of the brain that controls learning and reward seem to contribute to addiction. When you receive a reward, either internal (such as a pleasurable sensation or benefit) or external, you are more likely to repeat the behaviour, which encourages learning. Initially, people use legal and illegal drugs because they bring benefits, such as enhancing enjoyment, taking the edge off stress or helping them cope with difficulties.

The brain's addiction pathway

Addiction is linked to changes in a part of the brain called the mesocorticolimbic pathway, which you use to learn what's good to eat and drink, what activities bring you pleasure and so on. The pleasurable 'reward' you get when you activate the pathway – the sensation of a sweet bar of chocolate, for example – means that you're more likely to try that again. In other words, you learn. Numerous rewarding stimuli, from sugar-laden foods to heroin to nicotine, increase the activity of this pathway. The pathway is overactive in people with addictions, which means that the learnt compulsion drives their drug use or excessive eating long after the pleasure's gone. If you abuse drugs speak to your GP, contact your local drug treatment services (<www.talktofrank.com/need-support>) or call the Frank drugs helpline on 0800 776600.

Memories associated with these rewards develop into internal drives that motivate and perpetuate the behaviour you've learnt.[10] That's why former smokers often experience intense cravings in circumstances and places – so-called cues – when and where they used to light up. In some cases, cravings for drugs (including cocaine, heroin, alcohol and nicotine) induced by cues increase over time after quitting.[11] This helps explains why smokers and other addicts sometimes relapse even after many years' abstinence.

Smoking

Nicotine, the addictive chemical in tobacco, and the plant's scientific name (*Nicotiana tabacum*), 'honour' Jean Nicot de Villemain (1530–1600), a sixteenth-century French ambassador to Portugal. Villemain introduced tobacco to Parisian society when he returned from Lisbon in 1561. Smoking rapidly became fashionable.

However, concerns that smoking harmed health soon emerged. In 1604, James I of England (James VI of Scotland) described smoking as 'loathsome to the eye, hateful to the nose, harmful to the brain, and dangerous to the lungs'. The German physician Samuel Thomas von Sömmering noted a link between pipe smoking and lip cancer in 1795.[12] We now know that smoking caused 86 per cent of lung cancers in the UK in 2010 as well as, among other malignancies: 65 per cent of cancers in the mouth, throat and oesophagus; 29 per cent of pancreatic cancers; and 22 per cent of stomach cancers.[13]

So, smoking's increasing social unacceptability – just look at the huddles of smokers outside offices, pubs and restaurants – is good news for our health. During the 1940s, about 70 per cent of men and 40 per cent of women smoked. Government statistics suggest that the proportion declined to 22 per cent of men and 20 per cent of women in England in 2009. Nevertheless, about 8.8 million people still risk their lives by smoking:

- Around half of those who do not quit smoking die prematurely from their addiction.
- Smokers are roughly twice as likely to die from cancer as non-smokers.
- Smoking increases the likelihood of suffering a stroke up to three-fold.
- Smoking underlies a fifth of deaths among middle-aged people.
- Smoking causes around half of all cases of heart disease.

On the other hand, quitting reduces your likelihood of developing most smoking-related diseases. According to the Department of Health, an average lifelong smoker dies about ten years sooner than would otherwise be the case. A person who stops smoking at 30 or 40 years of age gains, on average, ten and nine years of life respectively. Even a 60-year-old gains three years by quitting.

The dangers to your family

If the benefits to your health are not enough to make you quit, think of the harm you're doing to your loved ones. Second-hand smoke contains more than 4,000 chemicals, including about 50 carcinogens – cancer-causing agents. This chemical cocktail increases the risk that people who inhale second-hand smoke will develop serious diseases, including cancer, heart disease, asthma and sudden infant death syndrome. For example, the risks that a woman who has never smoked will develop lung cancer and heart disease are 24 and 30 per cent greater, respectively, if she lives with a smoker.

Making quitting easier

On some measures, nicotine is more addictive than heroin or cocaine. As a result, fewer than 1 in 30 smokers quit each year and more than half relapse within a year, partly because of the intense withdrawal symptoms, which can leave you irritable, restless and anxious, experiencing insomnia and intensely craving a cigarette. The good news is that these generally abate over two weeks or so.

If you can't tough it out, nicotine replacement therapy (NRT) 'tops up' levels in the blood, without exposing you to the other harmful chemicals. So, NRT can alleviate the withdrawal symptoms and increase your chances of quitting by between 50 and 100 per cent. You can chose from various types of NRT. Patches reduce withdrawal symptoms over a relatively long time, but have a slow onset of action. Nicotine chewing gum, lozenges, inhalers and nasal spray act more quickly. Talk to your pharmacist or GP to find the right combination for you. Doctors can prescribe other treatments, such as bupropion and varenicline. While these offer a helping hand, you still need to be motivated to quit.

Tips to help you quit

In addition to NRT, a few simple hints may make life easier:

- Set a quit date, when you will stop completely. Smokers are more likely to quit if they set a specific date rather than saying, for example, that they'll give up in the next two months.
- Quit abruptly. People who cut back the number of cigarettes they smoke usually inhale more deeply to get the same amount of nicotine. Nevertheless, cutting back seems to increase the likelihood that you will eventually quit by, in some studies, 70 per cent compared with those who never cut back. So, while reduction takes you a step towards kicking the habit, don't stop there.
- Plan ahead: For a couple of weeks before you quit, keep a diary of problems and situations that tempt you to light up, such as stress, coffee, meals, pubs or work breaks. Understanding when and why you light up helps you find alternatives or avoid the cue.
- Try to find something to take your mind off smoking. If you find yourself smoking when you get home in the evening, try a new hobby or exercise. If you find car journeys boring without a cigarette, try an audio book. Most people find that the craving for a cigarette usually only lasts a couple of minutes.

- Smoking is expensive. Keep a note of how much you save and spend at least some of it on something for yourself.
- Tackle stress: Try 'active relaxation' (page 80) or exercise, or take part in a hobby that you enjoy.
- Ask if your area offers NHS anti-smoking clinics, which provide advice, support and, when appropriate, NRT. You can also obtain a free 'quit smoking' support pack from the NHS Smoking Helpline (0800 022 4332).
- Hypnosis can increase the chances of quitting smoking almost five-fold according to an analysis of four studies.[14] Ask your doctor for a recommendation or contact the British Association of Medical Hypnosis.

You might also need to deal with hunger pangs. Military commanders from the Thirty Years War to the First World War encouraged smoking to blunt fear and hunger. But try to avoid reaching for the sweet packet – which may mean you put weight on. In one study, people who quit smoking without treatment gained, on average, 1.12 kg during the month after quitting and 4.67 kg after a year.[15] However, 16 per cent of people *lost* weight after quitting and 37 per cent gained less than 5 kg. Only 13 per cent gained more than 10 kg.[15] Try the weight loss tips on page 71. If you really crave sugar, try sweet fruits, such as dates, kiwi fruit and pineapple.

Dealing with setbacks

Nicotine is incredibly addictive and, not surprisingly, Russell points out, most smokers make three or four attempts to quit before they succeed. Regard any relapse as a temporary setback, set another quit date and try again. It is also worth trying to identify why you relapsed. Were you stressed out? If so, why? Was smoking linked to a particular time, place or event? Once you know why you slipped you can develop strategies to stop the problem in the future. So, as the old health promotion advertisement suggests, 'Don't give up on giving up.'

Drinking

Heavy drinking isn't confined to youths sprawled senselessly drunk on the streets. According to the Office for National Statistics, in 2011, 38 per cent of people in managerial and professional households drank more than the recommended limit (four units for men, three units for women) on at least one day in the previous week. This compares to 28 per cent in 'routine' work or manual work households. Furthermore, 19 per cent and 15 per cent respectively drank harmful amounts of alcohol (eight units for men, six units for women) on at least one day in the previous week.

A UK unit of alcohol

A UK unit of alcohol contains 8 g alcohol. So:

- Half a pint of normal strength beer, lager or cider equals one unit.
- One small (100 ml) glass of wine equals one unit.
- A large (175 ml) glass of wine equals two units.
- A single (25 ml) measure of spirits equals one unit.
- One 275 ml bottle of alcopop (5.5 per cent/volume) equals 1.5 units.

Some studies and websites refer to an American 'drink', which contains 14 g of alcohol or just less than two British units.

A toast to good health?

The rising tide of liver disease and the burden imposed by alcohol-related injuries on already stretched casualty departments eloquently testify to the harm caused by excessive drinking. Indeed, a quarter of admissions to intensive care units in Scotland in 2009 were alcohol related.[16]

However, many health problems emerge only after years of heavy drinking. For example, excessive alcohol consumption causes around 1 in every 25 cancers,[17] including those of the mouth and throat, oesophagus (food pipe), colon (large bowel), rectum, larynx (voice box), liver and breast.[18]

But the liver, which breaks alcohol down, bears the brunt of the ill effects. Almost all men who usually drink more than 40–80 g of alcohol a day (5 to 10 units) for between 10 and 12 years develop alcoholic liver disease. In women, consuming more than 20–40 g a day (2.5 to 5 units) for 10 to 12 years makes alcoholic liver disease almost inevitable.[19] The risk of developing cirrhosis (potentially health-damaging liver scarring) doubles if you drink more than 50 g alcohol daily (about six units) and increases approximately five-fold among those drinking more than 100 g a day for several years.[20] Overall, alcohol accounts for more than a third (37 per cent) of deaths from liver disease, according to a 2012 report from the National End of Life Care Intelligence Network.

To look at the death toll another way: liver disease accounts for around 1 in10 deaths among people in their 40s – and alcohol abuse causes most of the mortality. Indeed, the death toll far exceeds the number of people killed by illegal drugs. In 2010, alcohol abuse killed 8,790 people in the UK – equivalent to a jumbo jet crashing every 20 days.

Heavy drinkers do not just harm themselves – alcohol abuse can irreconcilably damage unborn children, destroy families or cause accidents that injure or kill others. If you know someone who is abusing alcohol you should – gently and sympathetically – advise them to seek help.

The dangers of drinking during pregnancy

Drinking excessively during pregnancy can cause foetal alcohol syndrome (FAS), which is characterized by hallmark abnormalities, such as a smooth cleft from the nose to upper lip, abnormalities in the gap between the upper and lower eyelids, a thin upper lip and impaired growth and mental problems. The National Organisation for Foetal Alcohol Syndrome (NOFAS-UK) suggests that 6,000–7,000 children are born in Britain each year with FAS and related milder versions of the ailment – roughly 1 per cent of babies. The NHS suggests that pregnant women and those trying to conceive should avoid alcohol. At most, you should drink one or two units once or twice a week.

Am I drinking excessively?

To stop you damaging your health, the NHS recommends not regularly drinking more than three to four units a day if you are a man or two to three units daily if you are a woman. (Regularly means every day or most days.) Obviously, if you have a health problem or are pregnant, you should follow your doctor's advice: your limit may differ from the government's recommendation.

So, how can you tell if you are abusing alcohol? Doctors can use several questionnaires to detect alcohol abuse, including the CAGE questionnaire. You may have an alcohol problem if you answer 'yes' to two or more of these questions:

C: Have you ever felt you should cut down on your drinking?
A: Have people annoyed you by criticizing your drinking?
G: Have you ever felt bad or guilty about your drinking?
E: Eye opener: Have you ever had a drink first thing in the morning to steady your nerves or to get rid of a hangover?

However, CAGE is not perfect. The 'ever' phrase means that the questionnaire captures people who had a drink problem but now abstain or drink safely. The Alcohol Use Disorders Identification Test (AUDIT) is a more detailed questionnaire (see <www.patient. co.uk/doctor/Alcohol-Use-Disorders-Identification-Test-(AUDIT). htm>). But don't leave it too late: most people tend to deny that they abuse alcohol until health, social or legal problems emerge.

Tips to cut down

Most people want to try to tackle problem drinking themselves before seeing a doctor or joining a support group such as Alcoholics Anonymous. The first step is to keep a diary of how much you drink and when (places and circumstances – such as when you're feeling down or stressed out) over a month or so. You need to note how much you drink and not just guess. According to a report published by Alcohol Concern in 2009, the average adult drinker underestimates consumption by the equivalent of a bottle of wine each week (a 750 ml bottle of 12 per cent wine contains nine units). You may find that the act of keeping track means that you start cutting down. If you get so drunk that you cannot recall how much you drank the night before, you almost certainly have a problem.

Your drinking pattern offers another clue. Most people vary their drinking pattern. People who abuse alcohol tend to drink more regularly, partly because they need to stave off withdrawal symptoms. Withdrawal symptoms typically peak between 24 and 48 hours after the last drink and can include shakes, insomnia, agitation, depression and seizures. Returning to your old pattern after abstaining for a while is common among people who abuse alcohol.

You should set a goal (but if you suffer from a serious disease speak to your doctor). Some people who drink heavily will need to abstain, probably for the rest of their life. However, other people find that they can cut back and drink within the recommended limit – but they need to remain alert for changes in their drinking habits.

Some people pick a day and decide that they'll stop or dramatically cut down. However, even if you plan to return to drinking safe levels of alcohol, it is worth 'drying out' and not drinking for at least a month to allow your body a chance to recover. (If you can't stop drinking for a few weeks, you might have an alcohol problem.) Other people find that it is easier to gradually reduce the amount they drink. So, it is important to keep using your diary to track your progress and help avoid any slips.

Whether or not to tell your family, friends and colleagues that you are trying to cut down on alcohol can be difficult. Some family

Simple tricks to cut back on drinking

Various tricks can help you reduce your consumption of alcohol:

- Replace large glasses with smaller ones.
- Use a measure to tell how many units of gin you're adding to your tonic or fingers of whisky you're pouring at home.
- Only drink alcohol with a meal.
- Look at the label and avoid wine with alcohol by volume (ABV) of 14 per cent or 15 per cent. Try to buy bottles containing around 10 per cent ABV instead.
- Alternate alcoholic beverages with water or soft drinks. This slows alcohol consumption and helps avoid dehydration.
- Mix your drink – try spritzers and shandies rather than wine and beer.
- Quench your thirst with a soft drink rather than an alcoholic beverage.
- Make sure you have 'dry' (drink-free) days each week. The power of cues means that you may need to avoid your usual haunts and drinking partners on dry days.
- Find a hobby that does not involve drinking.
- When you're out with a large group, buying rounds can rapidly rack up the amount you consume. The group tends to keep pace with the fastest drinker. Try to buy rounds only when you're in small groups.
- Have soft drinks between the alcoholic drinks. You can ask for bottles of beer, shandies and spritzers, or halves instead of pints.
- Eat before you start drinking and regularly have snacks. Food slows the speed at which you will absorb alcohol.

and friends offer advice and support. Others may feel that you are challenging their drinking habits – and may prove hostile or condescending, especially if some of your social life or occupation revolves around drinking. In such cases, offer to be the designated driver or tell a white lie and claim that you're on medication and your doctor has advised you not to drink.

If you just can't quit

Several books and websites can help you reduce your drinking. If you feel you really can't quit without help, your doctor can refer you to NHS alcohol services or offer drugs to help you deal with cravings, as well as 'talking therapies' and counselling that will help you understand why you drink, how to cut down and the best way to deal with any difficult situations. For example, if you rely on a nightcap to get to sleep try the tips on page 94. If you drink to cope with pain, your doctor can suggest alternative painkillers. Some people abuse alcohol because they are depressed, anxious or suffer from another psychiatric illness. Furthermore, Alcoholics Anonymous and other support groups help many people – although they're not for everyone. As we've seen (page 38), some people find that taking part in formal religious activities helps them overcome alcohol and drug abuse.

If you find cutting down tough, you should ask yourself some searching questions. You could even keep a diary to record your thoughts (although I would suggest you keep it to yourself). People start drinking because alcohol offers benefits – maybe in social situations or to unwind. Writing a narrative – such as a story that reflects your experience or a diary – helps you identify triggers and cues: circumstances, places and emotions that you associate with drinking. So, walking past your local can trigger an urge for a pint or a meal in a favourite restaurant can trigger a desire for a bottle of wine. Obviously, avoid these cues as far as possible. And if stress triggers your drinking, try to bolster your defences, with meditation, exercise and so on.

Alcohol is such a part of most people's everyday life that it is easy to underestimate the harm that excessive drinking causes, the numbers of lives it damages, the pain it causes. Some diseases may mean you need to become teetotal. If not, you need to ensure you keep your consumption in check – for the sake of your health holistically.

The healthy alternative

Instead of alcohol, drink plenty of water and herbal teas. Even mild dehydration can cause a variety of unpleasant symptoms including: reduced vigilance and concentration; poor memory; increased tension or anxiety; fatigue and headache.[21, 22, 23] One study included 102 patients who experienced at least two moderately intense headaches (such as tension headaches and migraine) or at least five mildly intense headaches per month and drank less than 2.5 litres of fluid daily. The researchers asked 52 patients to increase the amount of water they drank by 1.5 litres a day.[23]

After three months, patients who increased the amount of water they drank showed better quality of life than the other patients ('controls'). Almost half (47 per cent) of those who increased water consumption reported 'much improvement' in their headaches compared to a quarter (25 per cent) of controls, although drinking more water did not change the number of days that patients experienced at least moderate headaches. So, try boosting your water consumption if you suffer regular headaches.[23]

The NHS notes that adults should drink 1.2 litres (six to eight glasses of water) each day to replace fluids they lose in urine, sweat and so on. If you feel thirsty for long periods, you're not drinking enough. And increase your intake during exercise or hot weather, if you feel lightheaded, pass dark-coloured urine or haven't passed urine within six hours. If you regularly feel thirsty despite maintaining your fluid intake, you should see your doctor. Excessive thirst can be a symptom of diabetes.

Healthy eating

Humans did not evolve to chomp on 'junk food' high in sugar and fat, and low in essential nutrients. Rather than sweets, cakes, pastries, take-away food and ready-meals, we evolved to eat a diet rich in fruit and vegetables and low in animal fats. In contrast, the typical modern Western diet produces an overabundance of energy. If you do not burn this energy off, the body stores the surplus in 'fat cells' as a precaution against famine. People living in industrialized nations can easily access food. As a result, about three-fifths of women and two-thirds of men in the UK are overweight or obese.

Weighty health problems

Excess weight causes or contributes to numerous serious ailments including heart disease, type 2 diabetes mellitus and about 1 in 18 cancers in the UK.[24] Furthermore, if current trends continue, another 11 million adults in the UK will be obese by 2030, resulting in 331,000 extra cases of coronary heart disease and strokes, 545,000 more cases of diabetes and 87,000 additional cancers.

On the other hand, a healthy diet can improve your holistic health. Changing your diet can seem daunting. But many people find that it takes only a month or so of eating – or not eating – a food for the change to become a habit. Indeed, some people (myself among them) who switch full-fat for skimmed milk soon find that they dislike the taste of full-fat milk. Similarly, many people soon lose their sweet tooth or taste for salt.

Free radicals

A slice of apple left exposed to the air soon turns brown. A group of tissue-damaging chemicals called free radicals causes the colour change. In the body, free radicals can damage tissues, cells and even our genetic code. Unfortunately, free radicals are all around us. Our body generates free radicals during the chemical reactions that keep us healthy. Our immune system uses free radicals to destroy invading bacteria. Pollution, cigarette smoke, pesticides and sunlight can generate free radicals.

So why are free radicals so dangerous? You may know that, put rather simply, electrons orbit the nucleus of an atom, rather like planets orbit a star. Electrons are most stable in pairs. As a result, a molecule or atom with a 'spare' electron – a free radical – will try to restore balance by 'stealing' an electron. This damages the 'donor' – such as fat, DNA or protein – and may even kill the cell. That's why free radicals seem to increase the risk of several serious illnesses, including heart disease, cancer, stroke, Alzheimer's disease and rheumatoid arthritis.

Salt

Almost everyone eats too much salt. High levels of salt (sodium chloride) in your blood can damage your cells. So, your body retains fluid to dilute the salt, which increases your blood pressure.

That means that a high salt intake makes it more likely you will develop hypertension, which can lead to stroke, heart disease and kidney damage.

The British Dietetic Association (BDA) comments that the average adult in the UK eats around 8.6 g of salt a day – about two teaspoons. The recommended intake for 'healthy' adults is 6 g of salt a day. But you should follow your doctor's advice: some people (e.g. those with liver disease, heart failure or hypertension) need to eat even less than this. To cut your salt intake:

- avoid foods – such as smoked meat and fish – that are high in salt;
- add as little salt as you can during baking and cooking;
- banish the salt cellar from the table;
- ask restaurants and take-aways for 'no salt';
- check levels of added salt and fat for 'self-basting' poultry;
- look for low-salt ketchup, pickles, mustard, yeast extract, stock cubes and so on;
- try using herbs, spices, chopped chillies and lime or lemon juice to give grains and other 'blander' foods more taste.

Watch for hidden salt

It is easy to tell that some snacks are salty. But many foods contain 'hidden salt': your taste buds will not set the alarm bells ringing. For example, manufacturers add surprisingly large amounts of salt to some soups, bread, biscuits and breakfast cereals. Indeed, salt already added to food accounts for three-quarters of our daily consumption. So, make sure you read the label and try to stick to low-salt foods.

The BDA advises choosing meals and sandwiches with less than 0.5 g sodium (1.25 g salt) per meal. Choose individual foods – such as soups and sauces – with less than 0.3 g sodium (0.75 g)

Table 4.2 Salt levels in food

Level	Salt content	Sodium content
High	More than 1.5 g per 100 g	More than 0.6 g per 100 g
Medium	0.3 g to 1.5 g per 100 g	0.1 g to 0.6 g per 100 g
Low	0.3 g or less per 100 g	0.1 g or less per 100 g

Source Adapted from the British Dietetic Association

per serving. Some labels list sodium, rather than salt. To convert sodium to salt, multiply by 2.5. So, 0.4 g of sodium is 1 g of salt. You can convert salt to sodium by dividing by 2.5 (see Table 4.2).

Fighting the fat

Despite numerous health warnings, too many of us still eat too much fat – one reason why our waistbands are bulging. Fat is the most concentrated energy source in our diet: 1 g provides nine calories. So, reducing fat aids weight reduction and helps you avoid heart disease, type 2 diabetes and some cancers.

Controlling cholesterol

Despite its bad press, cholesterol is essential for holistic health. Cholesterol is a building block of the membranes in every cell. Cholesterol helps form the myelin sheath that surrounds many nerves and ensures signals travel properly. And cholesterol forms the backbone of several hormones – including oestrogen, testosterone and progesterone – that carry messages around our bodies.

But poor diets and a lack of exercise (which burns up fat) mean that many of us have too much of a good thing. Nevertheless, the amount of cholesterol in your blood depends more on the saturated fat than the cholesterol in your diet. Indeed, few foods – with the exceptions of eggs, kidneys, prawns and liver – contain high levels of cholesterol. As a result, diet accounts for only around a third of the cholesterol in our bodies.

Types of fat

Broadly, foods contain two types of fat.

- Saturated fat comes mainly from animal sources, and is generally solid at room temperature.
- Unsaturated fat derives mainly from vegetables, nuts and seeds, and is usually liquid at room temperature. Olive oil is an unsaturated fat, for example. There are two main subtypes: monounsaturated and polyunsaturated fat. Fish is especially high in a particularly beneficial polyunsaturated fat (page 66).

Indeed, eggs are highly nutritious, which makes sense when you think how well they support growth. For example, eggs are rich in protein, vitamins A, B, D and E, zinc, iron and other minerals. It is fine to go to work on an egg (boiled or poached rather than fried), as part of a balanced diet.

Focus on saturated fat

Rather than worrying about cholesterol, focus on saturated fat. The liver converts saturated fat into cholesterol. The BDA notes that

Table 4.3 Foods high in saturated fat and low-fat alternatives

	Avoid	Low-fat alternative
Snacks	Crisps, savoury snacks cooked in oil	Fresh or dried fruit, handful of nuts
Fats for cooking and spreading	Lard, dripping, ghee, cream and butter	Olive, sunflower, soya or rapeseed (blended vegetable) oils, margarines and spreads
Meat	Processed food: sausages, burgers, pâté, salami, meat pies and pasties	Choose lean cuts of meat and mince (check labels or ask the butcher) Trim off fat – you can ask the butcher Skinless chicken and turkey Vegetarian options (lentils, chick peas and soya) Try Vegemince or soya mince instead of ground beef
Fish	Deep fried (e.g. take-away) fish and chips	Oily fish such as salmon, mackerel, sardines
Sauces	Creamy or cheesy sauces	Tomato or vegetable-based sauces
Dairy	Full-fat varieties	Skimmed (or at least semi-skimmed) milk; reduced-fat cheddar and low-fat yoghurt Try grating cheese or using a strong flavoured variety, which may mean you need to use less
Cooking	Pan or deep fry	Grill, steam or oven bake Avoid breadcrumbs that soak up fat

Source Adapted from the British Dietetic Association

most people in the UK eat about 20 per cent more than the recommended levels (no more than 20 g and 30 g of saturated fat a day for women and men respectively). So, most of us should eat more low-fat foods, which contain 1.5 g or less saturated fat per 100 g. High-fat foods contain more than 5 g of saturated fat per 100 g.

Table 4.3 suggests some ways you could cut your consumption of saturated fat. But remember that you're looking for a balanced diet. I'd be hard pressed to give up eating strong, full-fat cheeses, especially as I eat little red meat. Nevertheless, I watch the amount that I eat. And, although I'm not a vegetarian, I prefer vegetable curries and spaghetti Bolognese and lasagne made with Vegemince. If you find low-fat foods a little bland, try adding chillies, herbs or spices.

Protein

Making sure you eat enough protein is essential for holistic health in numerous ways, including:

- aiding growth and helping repair and regenerate your tissues;
- forming specialized proteins, including enzymes that speed up the chemical reactions that are essential for life;
- forming the scaffold that supports the cell's shape;
- making antibodies, which are essential for fighting infections.

The BDA suggests that the 'general sedentary population' should eat between 0.80 and 1.0 g of protein for each kilogram of their bodyweight each day. Endurance athletes (1.2–1.4 g per kg bodyweight) and strength athletes need slightly more (1.2–1.7 g per kg bodyweight per day). But while eating sufficient protein is essential for holistic health, it is important to get the balance right. For example:

- A high protein intake seems to increase the risk of colon cancer. So, the government recommends that healthy adults should not eat more than twice the recommended protein level.
- The National Osteoporosis Society points out that a protein-rich diet increases the acidity of the blood and other fluids in the body. (Proteins are made from long chains of amino acids.) The increased acidity tends to draw minerals, including calcium, from the bones, which weakens the skeleton. So, sticking to the recommended amount of protein may help keep your bones healthy.

- People who eat large amounts of red meat may be 24–36 per cent more likely to develop diabetes.[25]

Animal protein – such as meat, chicken and fish – can be loaded with saturated fat. So, choose the leanest cuts of meat and trim any visible fat. That's one reason why chicken helps you control your fat consumption: most of the fat is outside the muscle and easily removed. The rest of your protein should come from, for example, soya, yogurt, nuts, seeds, legumes and fish. Indeed, eating fish offers other holistic health benefits.

Fish and omega-3 fatty acids

Life inside the Arctic Circle is tough. As few plants survive, the traditional diet of first nation Arctic people consists of fish and animals that, in turn, eat marine life, such as seals. In the 1970s, for example, Greenland Inuits ate around 400 g of seafood a day.[26] Despite this meat-based diet, first nation Arctic people seem to be less vulnerable to several diseases – including diabetes, heart disease, arthritis and asthma – than people in 'industrialized' countries.

Table 4.4 Examples of fish and seafood high in omega-3 fatty acids

Anchovy

Black cod (sablefish)

Crab

Dogfish (rock salmon)

Halibut

Herring

Mackerel

Mussels

Oysters

Pilchards

Rainbow trout

Sardines

Salmon

Tuna (especially bluefin)

Source Adapted from the University of Michigan and the British Dietetic Association

Fish and, therefore, animals that survive on marine life are rich in omega-3 fatty acids, also called omega-3 polyunsaturated fatty acids (PUFA) and these account for much of the benefit offered by the Arctic diet. For example, heart attacks were ten times less common among Greenland Inuits than in people from Denmark. On average, Greenland Inuits ate 14 g of omega-3 fatty acids a day, the Danes just 3 g.[26] Eating fish once or twice a week (30 g to 60 g a day) reduces the risk of death from heart disease by between 30 and 60 per cent.[27] Furthermore, eating oily fish, the BDA points out, keeps joints healthy, while omega-3 PUFAs are important for memory, intellectual performance and healthy vision. Your mother was right: fish really is brain food.

We can make omega-3 fatty acids from another fat (alpha-lino-lenic acid) in green leafy vegetables, nuts, seeds and their oils. But it is a slow process. So, eating fish and seafood high in omega-3 PUFAs boosts levels of this essential nutrient. Table 4.4 lists examples of fish and seafood high in omega-3 fatty acids.

The BDA advises that adults and children over 12 years of age should eat two portions of fish per week (a portion is about 140 g once cooked). One of these meals should be an oily fish. Omega-3 PUFA levels are higher in fresh fish. If you're eating canned fish, check the label to make sure processing hasn't depleted the omega-3 oils. It is also worth trying to check that the fish comes from sustainable stocks (<www.fishonline.org>).

If at first you do not like the taste of oily fish, do not give up without trying some different fish and a few recipes. There are plenty of suggestions on the internet (e.g. <www.thefishsociety.co.uk>) and in cookbooks. For an island nation, our tastes in fish are remarkably conservative.

If you really cannot stomach the taste of oily fish, you could try a supplement. As I've stressed several times already, speak to your doctor first if you're taking other medicines or have a chronic disease. For example, if you have diabetes, you may need to avoid omega-3 supplements, which may increase blood sugar levels. Your doctor can also prescribe a highly concentrated version of omega-3 fatty acids.

Vegetables, fruit and fibre

Our ancestors picked plants, fished and hunted. They ate vegetables, legumes, fruits and whole grains, which were usually fresh, often raw. This traditional diet is high in fibre and rich in vitamins and other micronutrients.[28] Doctors and complementary therapists usually agree that limiting processed foods loaded with sugar, salt, preservatives, colourings and flavourings helps bolster your holistic health.

Boost your fibre intake

Dietary fibre (roughage) is the part of plants that humans cannot digest, such as the outer layers of sweetcorn, beans, wheat and corn. There are two main types of fibre:

- Insoluble fibre remains largely intact as it moves through your digestive system. However, insoluble fibre makes defecation easier.
- Soluble fibre dissolves in water in the gut, forming a gel which soaks up fats. So, you absorb less fat from a meal, lowering your blood cholesterol levels. Soluble fibre also releases sugar slowly, which helps stave off hunger pangs and so helps you lose weight.

Dieticians recommended that healthy adults should eat at least 18 g of fibre a day. Currently, the average UK adult eats about 14 g of fibre a day. So boost your consumption of: oats and oat bran; fruit and vegetables; nuts and seeds; pulses (such as peas, soya, lentils and chickpeas) and so on.

Whole grains

Whole grains are an especially rich source of fibre. Grains – the seeds of cereals, such as wheat, rye, barley, oats and rice – have three areas:

- Bran, the outer layer, is rich in fibre and packed with nutrients. Bran covers the 'germ' and endosperm.
- The germ develops into a new plant. So, the germ is packed with nutrients. Wheat germ, for example, contains high levels of vitamin E, folate (folic acid), zinc, magnesium and other vitamins and minerals.
- The central area (endosperm) is high in starch and provides the energy the germ needs to develop into a new plant.

Many food manufacturers refine grain by stripping off the bran and germ, and keeping the white endosperm. However, refining also strips off most of the nutritional value: whole grains contain up to 75 per cent more nutrients than refined cereals, the BDA points out. In addition to fibre, whole grains mop up tissue-damaging free radicals (page 61).

Regularly eating whole grains as part of a low-fat diet and a holistically healthy lifestyle cuts the risk of heart disease by up to 30 per cent. Furthermore, men who ate, on average, 10.2 g of cereal fibre a day were 30 per cent less likely to develop type 2 diabetes than those who ate 2.5 g a day. Women who consumed an average of 7.5 g of cereal fibre a day were 28 per cent less likely to develop diabetes than women who ate 2 g a day.[25]

Despite these benefits, 95 per cent of adults in the UK do not eat enough whole grains. Nearly a third do not eat any. The BDA advocates getting at least half your starchy carbohydrates from whole grains (two to three servings daily). Try eating more foods with 'whole' in front of the grain's name – such as wholewheat pasta and whole oats.

Five portions of fruit and vegetables

Fruit and vegetables are rich in vitamins, minerals and fibre – which is why you should eat five portions a day. A portion weighs about 80 g. Cooking can leach nutrients from fruits and vegetables. So, either eat fruit raw or cook vegetables using a small amount of unsalted water for the shortest time you can. Lightly steaming and

Table 4.5 Examples of a portion of fruit and vegetables

One medium-sized fruit (banana, apple, pear, orange)
One slice of a large fruit (melon, pineapple, mango)
Two smaller fruits (plums, satsumas, apricots, peaches)
A dessert bowlful of salad
Three heaped tablespoons of vegetables
Three heaped tablespoons of pulses (chickpeas, lentils, beans)
Two to three tablespoons ('a handful') of grapes or berries
One tablespoon of dried fruit
One glass (150 ml) of unsweetened fruit or vegetable juice or smoothie (two or more glasses of juice a day still counts as only one portion)

stir-frying are healthy alternatives. And scrub rather than peel potatoes, carrots and so on: the skin often contains valuable nutrients. Table 4.5 gives some examples of a portion of fruit or vegetables.

Seeds, nuts and legumes

Seeds, nuts and legumes are an excellent source of fibre and other nutrients. However, plants use energy stored in seeds to aid the plant's early growth and development. So, they're relatively high in calories.

Not all 'nuts' are, strictly, nuts. Brazil and cashew nuts are seeds, for example. Peanuts are legumes, more closely related to peas and lentils than chestnuts and hazel nuts. You can ponder such botanical quibbles while eating a handful of almonds, cashews, walnuts, Brazils and pecans a day as snacks, with cereal and in baking.

Legumes are a cheap source of protein, are high in fibre and help control levels of fats in the blood. So, try to eat more:

- baked beans (although watch the sugar and salt in some brands)
- kidney beans
- chickpeas – try a chickpea dahl, for example
- red and green lentils
- mung beans
- butter beans
- black beans
- split peas – pease pudding is one of my favourite foods, cheap and nutritious
- haricot beans
- soya beans, which are rich in polyunsaturated fats and low in saturated fat. The BDA notes that one portion of soya beans counts towards your five portions of fruits and vegetables a day. So, try soya milk, tofu, tempeh, miso and so on.

Vegetarian cookbooks are full of ideas to boost your bean consumption. You can also add beans to 'bulk' up stews if you're cutting down on meat.

Dieting to lose weight

Weight itself is not a very good guide to your risk of developing diseases linked to excess body fat. Weighting 14 stone is fine if you're 6 foot 5. But you'd be seriously obese if you're 5 foot 6.

Table 4.6 Waist sizes linked to health risk

	Health at risk	Health at high risk
Men	Over 94 cm (37 inches)	Over 102 cm (40 inches)
Women	Over 80 cm (32 inches)	Over 88 cm (35 inches)
South Asian men		Over 90 cm (36 inches)
South Asian women		Over 80 cm (32 inches)

Source Adapted from the British Heart Foundation

Body mass index (BMI) takes your height and weight into account and so offers a better indication of whether you're overweight (for an easy way to calculate your BMI, see <www.nhs.uk/Tools/Pages/Healthyweightcalculator.aspx>). You should try to keep your BMI between 18.5 and 24.9 kg/m². Below this and you're dangerously underweight. A BMI between 25.0 and 29.9 kg/m² suggests that you are overweight. You're probably obese if your BMI exceeds 30.0 kg/m². However, BMI may overestimate body fat in athletes, body builders and other muscular people (such as hod carriers). On the other hand, BMI may underestimate body fat in older persons and people who have lost muscle.

Doctors and gyms can use a monitor to check your body fat. However, not all fat is equal. Abdominal obesity damages your health more than fat elsewhere in your body, especially in people of South Asian descent. So, waist size can tell you whether your health is at risk (see Table 4.6).

Tips to help you lose weight

Many of us need to shed a few pounds as part of our holistic drive towards health and well-being. Unfortunately, losing weight is not easy – whatever the latest fad diets would have you believe. After all, millions of years of evolution drive us to consume food in times of feast to help us survive times of famine. And you can't stop eating as you can quit smoking or drinking alcohol. However, the following tips may help:

- Keep a food diary and record everything you eat and drink for a couple of weeks. It is often easy to see where you inadvertently pile on the extra calories: the odd biscuit here, the extra glass of wine or a full-fat latte there. It soon adds up. A food diary can also help you see if you are eating fatty or high-salt food.

- Set a realistic, specific target. Rather than saying that you want to lose weight, resolve to lose two stone. Use the BMI to set your target weight. Cutting your intake by between 500 and 1,000 calories each day can reduce bodyweight (assuming your BMI is stable) by between 0.5 and 1.0 kg each week.[28] Steadily losing around a pound or two a week reduces your chances of putting it back on again.
- Think about how you tried to lose weight in the past. What techniques and diets worked? Which failed to make a difference or proved impossible to stick to? Did going to a support group help?
- Do not let a slip-up derail your diet. Try to identify why you indulged. What were the triggers? A particular occasion? Do you comfort eat? Once you know why you slipped you can develop strategies to stop the problem in the future.
- Begin your diet when you are at home over a weekend or a holiday and you do not have a celebration (such as Christmas or a birthday) planned. It is tougher changing your diet on a Monday morning or when you're away on business in a hotel faced with fat-laden food, caffeine-rich drinks and alcohol.

If this fails, talk to your GP or pharmacist. Several medicines may help kick-start your weight loss. You can also try cognitive behavioural therapy (CBT – see page 84) and hypnosis. CBT can reduce weight by around 6 lb (2.75 kg). Adding hypnosis (page 77) to CBT can increase weight loss to almost 15 lb (6.75 kg).[14] None of these approaches offers a magic cure and you will still need to change your lifestyle. However, they help put you on the right course towards weight loss and better holistic health.

5

Complementary therapy: supporting your inner healer

As we've seen, modern medicine rarely fully addresses a disease's spiritual, emotional and psychological aspects – many of which impose heavy burdens on patients. In contrast, complementary medicine promotes a holistic view addressing an illness's diverse causes and consequences.[1] Complementary therapies do not replace mainstream treatment. Rather, complementary therapies control symptoms, improve well-being, enhance quality of life, bolster a healthy lifestyle and may augment conventional treatments' efficacy. However, never stop a treatment or reduce a drug's dose without speaking to your doctor.

Unfortunately, we can only skim the surface of this vast area – numerous books cover the various options suitable for a particular condition. Nevertheless, the examples in this chapter illustrate that complementary therapies can help you derive the most benefit from conventional care, restore your control over your illness and help your quest for holistic health.

A popular approach

Their holistic perspective helps account for complementary therapies' continuing popularity despite modern medicine's remarkable successes. For example, between 17 and 78 per cent of people with cancer (depending on the patients studied and the malignancy's stage) use at least one complementary therapy.[2] Around 1 in 10 heart disease patients in the West Midlands attending hospital for a check-up used complementary and alternative medicine.[3] A survey of asthma patients in England found that 15 per cent had used complementary therapies.[4]

In addition, many people use complementary therapies to prevent, rather than treat, disease or to alleviate stress and other minor ailments that they don't feel need a doctor's attention. Indeed, in 1998 almost 11 per cent of 2,669 adults surveyed in England had used at least one of the following: acupuncture, chiropractic, homeopathy, hypnotherapy, osteopathy or medical herbalism – equivalent to 22 million visits. When the researchers included reflexology and aromatherapy, as well as homeopathic or herbal remedies bought from chemists or health shops, the proportion rose to about 28 per cent. Overall, almost half (47 per cent) had used at least one of these complementary medicines at some time.[5]

Most people feel they benefit from complementary treatment. In one study, more than half said that the therapy always (23 per cent) or usually (33 per cent) helped their asthma. A further 28 per cent said that the complementary treatment sometimes helped. Fewer asthma symptoms (reported by 44 per cent) and helping to calm breathing and reduce panic (37 per cent) were the most commonly reported benefits.[4]

Courting controversy

Despite being popular and despite millions of people feeling they benefit, complementary medicines often attract considerable controversy, in part because traditional explanations fit uneasily with modern scientific medicine. For example, scientific studies show that acupuncture alleviates a range of ailments. However, few conventional Western doctors accept the traditional Chinese explanation that acupuncture balances the flow of chi (the life force) along 12 meridians (channels) that run throughout the body linking our organs and systems. Yet, as mentioned in Chapter 1, 'there is no accepted mechanism by which [acupuncture] could have persisting effects on chronic pain'.[6]

Cynics also point to the lack of evidence supporting many complementary therapies – acupuncture and certain herbal medicines are notable exceptions. Certainly, few complementary therapies undergo the same rigorous testing as modern medicines. However, as clinical trials are expensive and pharmaceutical companies fund most trials, this lack of studies is not surprising. Nevertheless, no evidence of effectiveness is not necessarily the same as evidence of no effect.

In addition, complementary therapists often combine approaches, which complicates disentangling the benefits of the various treatments. Naturopathy, for example, combines dietary changes (Chapter 4) and other approaches. In one study, researchers treated 41 people who experienced moderate to severe anxiety by using 'naturopathic care' consisting of dietary advice, deep breathing relaxation, a standard multi-vitamin, and the ayurvedic herbal medicine ashwagandha (*Withania somnifera*), also called Indian ginseng. Another 40 people were treated with psychotherapy ('talking therapies'), deep breathing relaxation techniques and placebo for the herbs and vitamins. After 12 weeks, scores on a questionnaire that measured anxiety showed a decline of approximately 57 per cent with naturopathic care and 31 per cent in those treated with psychotherapy. In addition, naturopathic care alleviated fatigue and improved mental health, concentration, social functioning, vitality and overall quality of life.[7]

Cynical healthcare professionals tend to dismiss complementary medicine's success as 'just placebo'. Yet as we've seen, the placebo response contributes to every medical intervention, whether conventional or complementary. In other cases, cynics ascribe the benefits to 'relaxation'. And relaxation certainly contributes. For example, Eileen Herzberg in *Thorsons Introductory Guide to Healing* cites the results of a survey that found that almost half of people felt 'deeply relaxed' and 41 per cent felt calm during a spiritual healing session. But relaxation is certainly not the whole story. Relaxation can't fully account for hypnotism's ability to counter the pain of an operation, for example (page 77).

Types of complementary medicine

Broadly, complementary medicines fall into one of four major types:

- Mind–body practices: these enhance integration between the brain, mind, body and behaviour. In the USA, deep breathing exercises are the most popular mind–body therapy (used by 12.7 per cent of adults in the year before the survey), followed by meditation (9.4 per cent), yoga (6.1 per cent), progressive muscle relaxation (2.9 per cent) and guided imagery (2.2 per cent). Less commonly used techniques included tai chi, qi gong, hypnosis and biofeedback.[1]

- Natural products, including herbs, vitamins, minerals and other supplements, such as omega 3 oils (page 66), glucosamine and chondroitin: many people take the latter two supplements to alleviate arthritis and other joint problems. Naturopathy and aromatherapy also use natural products.
- Manipulative and body-based complementary practices, such as massage, Alexander therapy, Shiatsu, chiropractic and osteopathy: these focus on bones, joints, muscles and so on.
- Other, including energy-field manipulation (e.g. crystal therapy, Reiki, Therapeutic Touch) and whole medicine systems, such as traditional Chinese, Arabic (Unani) and ayurvedic medicines, homeopathy and naturopathy.

In other words, there's a vast range of complementary treatments to choose from – and these approaches may overlap. Shiatsu practitioners may massage parts of the body to unblock the flow of chi. In other words, Shiatsu is both a manipulative and energy field therapy. Indeed, it's sometimes hard to see the boundary between mainstream and complementary therapy. Russell notes that ayurvedic medicine is mainstream in India, but is a complementary treatment in the UK. Given the proliferation of possible treatments, it's important to take advice from your doctor or patient group and to read up on the approach you want to try. It's worth making the effort: the following examples illustrate how complementary medicine can help as part of a holistic approach to health.

Biofeedback

Biofeedback allows you to exert some control over the autonomic nervous system (page 23), which usually works without conscious control. Biofeedback machines and software typically make a sound or show a display that varies according to the activity of your autonomic nervous system. You may monitor your heartbeat, for example. By listening to the sounds or watching the display, practitioners train themselves to regulate the signals. This allows them to exert some control over their autonomic functions, such as heartbeat, blood pressure, respiration rate and muscle tension.

There's strong evidence from scientific studies that biofeedback helps several diseases including urinary incontinence in women, anxiety, Attention Deficit Hyperactivity Disorder, chronic pain, constipation, epilepsy, headache, hypertension, motion sickness, Raynaud's disease and temporomandibular joint disorder. Temporomandibular joint disorder arises from problems with the muscles, joints and bones that control chewing; patients report pain in the head, neck, face, ear and head, a jaw that is locked in position or is difficult to open, problems biting, and 'clicking' or 'popping' when they bite.[1] Several commercial biofeedback machines and computer programmes are available.

Hypnosis

For centuries, conventional doctors dismissed hypnotism as a stage trick, its benefits confined to weak-willed, gullible people. In 1890, the *British Medical Journal* (*BMJ*) called hypnotism 'a dangerous mental poison, and as such it needs to be fenced round with as many restrictions as the traffic in other kinds of poison'. The *BMJ* added that hypnotism is 'fraught with many dangers to the nervous equilibrium and psychological soundness of the subject'.[8]

Some doctors even suggested that subjects 'faked' responses to please their hypnotist. Yet Bivins recounts the 'respectable' surgeon from Nottingham who, in 1842, used hypnotism (then called mesmerism) during an operation to amputate his patient's leg. At the time, alcohol offered the only anaesthetic and patients, not surprisingly, often needed to be drunk and tied down to allow the surgeon to operate. Around the same time, James Esdaile, a Scottish surgeon working near Calcutta, removed a scrotal tumour using hypnosis as anaesthesia. And in 1829, the French doctor Pierre-Jean Chapelain used hypnosis as an anaesthetic during mastectomy for breast cancer.[9] It is hard to believe someone would endure the pain of a scrotal operation, an amputation or a mastectomy to please the surgeon. The advent of powerful painkillers and anaesthetics meant that healers no longer resorted to hypnosis, but these examples underscore the power of hypnotism.

Today, doctors still don't fully understand how hypnotism works. Essentially, however, hypnosis is focused attention and concentration. Some hypnotists describe the process as similar to being 'so lost in a book or movie that it is easy to lose track of what is going on around you'.[9] And despite the cynicism of Victorian doctors – who probably worried that hypnotism could take some of their business – hypnosis helps with controlling pain, alleviating stress and changing harmful habits such as abusing alcohol, comfort eating (page 72) or smoking (page 54). In people with cancer, hypnosis can reduce fatigue, distress, pain, nausea and some side effects of treatment. For example, hypnotists can suggest that the person will experience less pain, be less bothered or can ignore the discomfort, or can replace pain with a numb or cool sensation.[9]

And hypnosis is safe. You won't lose control: a hypnotist can't make you do or say anything he or she wants. You'll be able to come 'out' of hypnosis whenever you want.[9] Some people also find that self-hypnosis helps. Numerous DVDs, CDs and books help you create the 'focused attention' that underpins hypnosis. Contact the British Association of Medical Hypnosis for further information.

Tai chi and qi gong

Meditation is not confined to sitting in the lotus position chanting 'om' or some other mantra. Tai chi, qi gong, yoga and Rosary prayer are all forms of meditation. However, learning classical meditation can be difficult without guidance. Many local adult education centres hold courses. Your church minister or spiritual adviser can educate you about the best way to pray.

Tai chi (*tai chi chuan*) is a 'soft' or 'internal' martial art that combines deep breathing, meditation and relaxation with sequences (called forms) of slow gentle movements that enhance fitness, strength and flexibility. This means that tai chi is often suitable (after checking with your doctor) for diseases as diverse as chronic obstructive pulmonary disease, Parkinson's disease and arthritis.

Tai chi may look undemanding until you try it. You can learn the tai chi short form in about 12 lessons. However, tai chi takes many years to master. Speeded up tai chi can offer effective self-defence – indeed, *chuan* means 'fist'. Speed up a raising hand and you may deflect a blow to the head, while a descending hand can deflect a kick.

Qi gong also combines deep breathing, meditation, relaxation and movements. However, the movements are more internally focused on the 'flow of energy' around the body than tai chi.[1] Contact the Tai Chi Union for Great Britain for more information.

Yoga

Yoga brings millions of people – from all religious backgrounds – inner peace, relief from stress and improved health. Yoga aims to harmonize consciousness, mind, energy and body. (The Indian root of yoga means 'to unite'.)

Essentially, yoga focuses on achieving controlled, slow, deep breaths, while the poses (asanas) increase fitness, strength and flexibility. As a result, yoga helps maintain suppleness of both body and mind (some of the poses require considerable concentration). Indeed, clinical studies suggest that yoga may help people with asthma, anxiety, headaches, depression, back and neck pain, fibromyalgia and chronic obstructive pulmonary disease.[10, 11] Yoga also improves mood and reduces anxiety more than the same time spent exercising by walking.[12]

Scientists are beginning to uncover the biological basis for yoga's benefits. For example, yoga down-regulates sympathetic nervous system activity and decreases cortisol, blood glucose, adrenaline and noradrenaline levels, heart rate, blood pressure and inflammation, as well as increasing levels of natural killer cells, part of our immune defences.[13] Contact the British Wheel of Yoga for more information.

Think about your breathing

One of the first things a yoga, martial arts or meditation teacher will probably tell you is that you are not breathing correctly. Most of us breathe shallowly, using the upper parts of our lungs. Try putting one hand on your chest and the other on your abdomen. Then breathe normally. Most people find that the hand on their chest moves while the one on the abdomen remains relatively still. To fill your lungs fully, try to make the hand on your abdomen rise, while keeping the one on the chest as still as possible.

Breathing deeply and slowly without gasping helps relaxation. If you feel stressed out try breathing in deeply through your nose for the count of four, hold your breath for a count of seven; then breathe out for a count of eight. Repeat a dozen times.

Active relaxation

There is nothing wrong with curling up with a good book or watching your favourite television programme. However, many of us need to take a more 'active' approach to relaxation.

As we've seen, relaxation down-regulates the sympathetic nervous system. So, for example, the National Institute for Health and Clinical Excellence (NICE) notes that relaxation therapies – including progressive muscle relaxation, meditation, yoga, assertiveness training and anger control techniques – reduce blood pressure by around 3.5 mmHg. A third of patients using these techniques show at least a 10 mmHg reduction in blood pressure. That's a similar amount to the improvement produced by many drugs for hypertension.

Furthermore, people with atopic dermatitis (allergic eczema) often experience intense itch. Around 80 per cent of patients report that stress exacerbates the itch. It's difficult to ignore the desire to scratch, which can damage the skin, intensify inflammation and exacerbate itch. In turn, the discomfort increases anxiety and stress. Relaxation therapies alleviate itch in part by tackling stress and anxiety, so breaking the cycle.[14] Clearly, relaxation and stress reduction more generally produce measurable biological benefits and, in turn, form an important part of the holistic approach to health and well-being.

Finding time to relax

The link between mind and body means that you cannot be mentally tense while your body is relaxed – which is one reason why laughter and tears alleviate tension and improve health (page 102) – or vice versa. Relaxing your body relaxes your mind.

The following tips should help you relax. You may need to adapt these if, for example, you want to meditate or practise yoga.

- Try to follow your relaxation therapy every day. Many people find that the early morning is the best for 'active relaxation'. The house is quiet and you will be better able to focus and less likely to drop off to sleep than later at night.
- Put yourself at your ease. Sit in a comfortable chair that supports your back. If you prefer, lie down. You might want to put cushions under your neck and knees. Take off your shoes, switch

off any bright lights and ensure the room is neither too hot nor too cold.

- Do not try to perform relaxation therapy on a full stomach. After a meal, blood diverts from your muscles to your stomach. Trying progressive muscle relaxation (see below) on a full stomach can cause cramps. And relaxation can make you more aware of your body's functions. A full stomach can be a distraction.
- Shut your eyes and, if it helps, play some relaxing music and burn some aromatherapy oils. One study, for example, found that the aroma of sweet orange reduces anxiety.[15]

Progressive muscular relaxation

Progressive muscular relaxation (PMR) aims to relax each part of your body in turn. To try PMR, put your hands by your side. Now clench your fists as hard as you can. Hold the fist for ten seconds. Now slowly relax your fist and let your hands hang loosely by your sides. Then shrug your shoulders as high as you can. Hold for ten seconds and then relax slowly. Now gently arch your back, hold for ten seconds and relax. Tense your muscles as you inhale. While you're tense, do not hold your breath. Try to breathe slowly and rhythmically. Exhale as you relax. Repeat each exercise three times, slowly, gently and gradually. Remember you're not body building, you're relaxing. Most PMR teachers advise mastering one muscle group at a time. So, it could take two or three months before you can tense and relax your entire body.

We become used to a certain amount of muscle tension. Our necks feel stiff. Our jaw muscles clench. We frown. But with practice, you will start recognizing when your muscles are tense during your everyday life – and you can then use PMR to relax the tense muscles. However, if you suffer from back problems, arthritis or any other serious medical disease or ailment, check with your doctor before trying PMR.

Your work environment and muscle tension

Poor posture at work can generate or exacerbate muscle tension. So, while sitting, try to keep your shoulders and head in a straight line and drop your shoulders. Sit upright at your desk with your feet on the floor. Arrange your computer keyboard so you can see it looking straight ahead without hunching or lifting your arms.

Herbalism: the foundation of modern drugs

Many complementary therapies – including hypnosis, herbalism and acupuncture – have heritages reaching back centuries before the advent of scientific medicine. For example, archaeologists uncovered sharpened stones that they believe were used for acupuncture dating from 10,000 BC. The first texts about acupuncture are more than 2,000 years old.

Herbalism predates even acupuncture – perhaps even before we became recognizably human. Chimpanzees and gorillas deliberately 'self-medicate' with plants active against parasites, often using the same herbs as local healers.[16] In 1960, archaeologists discovered a Neanderthal skeleton buried in caves in Shanidar, Iraq, with several plants used by modern herbalists – including cornflower, yarrow and groundsel – surrounding the remains. The plants probably formed part of the Neanderthals' pharmacy. Today, herbal and other treatments remain important worldwide: according to the World Health Organization, 80 per cent of the population in some Asian and African countries still depend on traditional medicine for health care.

When tradition trumps technology

Sometimes traditional medicine seems to owe more to superstition than to science. However, Bivins notes, traditional frameworks – even when as apparently bizarre as astrological correspondences, such as linking Jupiter with the liver or associating Saturn with bones – allowed doctors to recognize patterns, organize their knowledge and apply that collective wisdom to particular patients. And patients often benefited.

Malaria was the scourge of early Europeans visiting the tropics. In the early seventeenth century, explorers in South America learnt that the bark of the cinchona tree alleviated malarial fevers. At the time, physicians believed that a benevolent God placed a cure for an area's diseases in the local environments – such as dock leaves near stinging nettles.

Today, we know that a drug in the bark – quinine – kills the parasite that causes malaria. Nevertheless, whether you organize your knowledge on the basis of a belief in a benevolent God, a chemical's biological benefits or both, cinchona bark still works.

Indeed, over millennia, traditional healers accumulated an impressive wealth of knowledge. For example:

- The tsetse fly infects around 12,000 people annually in sub-Saharan Africa with the parasite that causes sleeping sickness, also called trypanosomiasis (*Trypanosoma brucei*). Scientists found that five plants traditionally used in Tanzania to treat sleeping sickness are effective against this devastating disease.[17]
- Bolivian traditional healers used Evanta (*Galipea longiflora*) to treat kala-azar and other difficult-to-treat diseases caused by another parasite (*Leishmania*). Scientists recently confirmed that *G. longiflora* kills *Leishmania* and possibly controls the chronic inflammation triggered by the parasite.[18]
- A Chinese herbal written between 281 and 340 BC suggests using a tea brewed from the leaves of sweet wormwood (*Artemisia annua*) for fevers and chills – malaria's hallmark symptoms. In 1972, Chinese scientists isolated the anti-malarial chemical artemisinin from sweet wormwood. Today, artemisinin often remains effective against the growing number of malaria parasites that are resistant to conventional treatments.[19]
- In 1763, the English chaplain Edward Stone found that willow bark alleviated ague, a fever caused by malaria, then rife in England. Aspirin is a chemically modified, less toxic version of the active ingredient in willow bark.
- In 1962, a botanist named Arthur Barclay peeled some bark from a Pacific yew tree (*Taxus brevifolia*) growing in the Gifford Pinchot National Forest in north-eastern USA. Oncologists now use a drug called paclitaxel, extracted from yew bark, to treat various malignancies including lung, breast and ovarian cancer.[20]

Using herbs safely

As these examples show, herbs can be potent. Indeed, certain herbs can interfere with conventional medicines, cause side effects or both. However, studying the safety of herbal treatments can prove difficult: plants contain a mixture of chemicals, several of which can contribute to the herb's benefits and adverse events. In *Health and Healing*, Andrew Weil notes, for example, that opium contains 22 active ingredients. To complicate matters further, many herbal formulations contain several different plants: some traditional

Chinese medicines contain more than 20 components. As herbs and other treatments may influence each other, assessing the benefits, side effects and interactions with conventional medicines can prove difficult.

On the other hand, the amount of biologically active chemicals in a herb is less than that in a conventional medicine. While this means that you are less likely to experience side effects, the benefits can take longer to emerge or may not be as marked. Nevertheless, if you develop any changes that could be side effects, stop taking the formulation and see your medical herbalist. And if you fail to experience any benefits after three months you should think about stopping the herb. Before you embark on a course of herbal supplements, speak to your doctor. Not all products include the detailed information you need to take the supplement safely.

If you decide to try herbal remedies or other supplements, make sure you buy reputable preparations from a shop with knowledgeable staff. You should also look for standardized extracts: the amount of active ingredient can vary depending where it is grown and when it is harvested. (That may be why some traditional herbals suggest gathering the plant at a particular time or associate the herb with a particular astrological sign.) Rather than treating yourself using herbs, it is best to consult a qualified medical herbalist and make sure to tell him or her about any disease or ailment or any conventional medicines you're taking.

Counselling and CBT

Sharing problems, asking for advice or a considering a different perspective often helps you overcome problems arising from a chronic disease or with life generally. Indeed, at least part of the benefit associated with religion probably arises from the spiritual leaders' often considerable counselling skills. The congregation or religious community often also draws on its collective experiences to help. Similarly, many people benefit from consulting counsellors and psychotherapists.

Counsellors and psychotherapists use a variety of 'talking therapies' to help you tackle your problems. One widely used approach, cognitive behavioural therapy (CBT), identifies the feelings, thoughts and behaviours associated with your disease or unhealthy lifestyle. You'll then question and test those feelings, thoughts, behaviours and beliefs, and will learn to replace unhelpful and unrealistic behaviours with approaches that actively address problems.

For example, CBT can use gradual exposure to feared situations or activities. So, a person with agoraphobia would spend increasing time in situations where escape might be difficult, such as travelling on public transport or visiting a shopping centre. Another element of CBT, called cognitive restructuring, replaces unhelpful and detrimental thoughts or anxieties with more positive thoughts. CBT usually uses explicit goals, often broken into manageable, short-term goals and supported by regular 'homework'.

Mindfulness

In some cases, therapists combine CBT with other approaches, such as mindfulness.[21] Definitions of mindfulness vary. But essentially mindfulness training encourages patients to concentrate, non-judgementally and openly, on the present rather than worry about what might happen or ruminate on the past. Some therapists compare mindfulness to waking up from life on automatic pilot. Mindfulness seems to increase your ability to regulate and manage behaviour as well as improving the flexibility of thinking, emotions and behaviour. As a result, people can adapt more effectively to life events.[22]

For example, a stress-reduction programme that encompasses mindfulness typically lasts between eight and ten weeks and may use meditation and yoga to help you recognize and escape from habitual, counterproductive thoughts and behaviours. So, used alongside CBT, mindfulness stress reduction helps people accept and tolerate the unpleasant emotions that the therapy or changing habitual behaviours may evoke.[22]

Mindfulness-based interventions alleviate a variety of ailments, including chronic pain, anxiety, depression, eating disorders, drug and alcohol abuse, and several other psychiatric conditions. Indeed, mindfulness-based CBT may reduce the risk that depression will relapse as effectively as antidepressants, in some patients at least.[22] Furthermore, eight weeks of mindfulness-based stress reduction therapy seems to reduce the intensity of inflammation provoked experimentally by applying a cream containing capsaicin – the active ingredient in chilli peppers – to the skin. Mindfulness's impact on inflammation was independent of the effect on stress.[23]

How effective is CBT?

Therapists use CBT to treat numerous problems, including depression, anxiety, insomnia, substance abuse and chronic pain. For example:

- Almost two-thirds (65 per cent) of back pain patients remain in pain after a year, according to a review of 11 studies.[24] Many patients with persistent low back pain believe that they cannot cope or cannot resume normal activities because they fear further injury. CBT targets such unhelpful coping strategies.[21]
- CBT can help adults with Attention Deficit Hyperactivity Disorder prioritize tasks, solve problems, change their environment to minimize distractions, and counter maladaptive thoughts.[25]
- Only around a third of people with depression respond adequately to antidepressants. A study of 469 adults in the UK who did not respond to antidepressants, 46 per cent of whom also underwent CBT, reported at least a 50 per cent reduction in depression after six months despite their poor response to antidepressants alone. This compared to 22 per cent of those managed with 'usual care', such as changing drugs or referring to psychiatric services.[26]
- Even DIY CBT works. In a study of 203 people in Glasgow, the severity of depression halved in 43 per cent of patients after four months of treatment with a self-help book and, on average, two face-to-face support sessions each lasting about 40 minutes. In comparison, only 26 per cent of those receiving usual care reported a halving in symptom severity. Overall, following the advice in the self-help book approximately doubled the chances of recovery from depression after four months and the benefits seemed to persist for at least a year.[27]

To discuss whether CBT or one of the other talking therapies could help you, contact the British Association for Counselling and Psychotherapy or ask your doctor's surgery if they can recommend a local counsellor.

Complementary therapy and holistic health

If you want to try complementary therapy as part of a holistic approach to health and well-being, check with your doctor first, especially if you have a chronic illness. Then ensure that you consult a registered practitioner, such as one recognized by the General Regulatory Council for Complementary Therapies or the Complementary and Natural Healthcare Council. Read up on the approach you are planning to use and make sure you understand the risks and benefits.

Keep a watch for side effects. For example, some alternative healers believe that complementary therapies drive out the toxins that have accumulated in your body. This toxic 'tsunami' can produce a detox 'crisis', characterized by unpleasant symptoms including headaches, fatigue and abdominal discomfort. In some cases, the healer and the person undergoing detox can dismiss adverse events as a crisis. So, you need to be careful if you experience any unexpected symptoms.

And you need to check that the treatments works. As mentioned before, one of the best ways is to keep a diary noting the symptoms, triggers and how you feel. If you don't feel any benefit after three months, discuss whether it is worth continuing your treatment with the practitioner.

6

Your companions for health

John Donne famously commented that 'no man is an island' and Polkinghorne remarks that human nature 'is partly constituted and expressed through a network of contacts with other persons'. Meals, for example, can be social events that help create and maintain social networks in the family and augment the benefits of a healthy diet. Indeed, social networks and mutual aid are basic biological drives: numerous animal species support other members of a 'kin' that share genes. And we don't even restrict altruism to humankind: companion animals – pets – can be invaluable partners on our road to recovery and enhance our health.

In addition, social networks can have a profound impact on our well-being in part by offering emotional and practical support. For instance, most people discuss their health with family, friends and colleagues. Indeed, Russell notes that between 70 and 90 per cent of health care takes place without the support of a folk or professional healer. But make sure you check their advice (page 12).

Paws for thought

We're a nation of animal lovers. British people own 10.3 million cats and 10.5 million dogs – not to mention millions more birds, rabbits, rodents, reptiles, fish and horses. And some bonds are remarkably strong. Indeed, we've lived side by side with dogs for perhaps more than 30,000 years.[1] Over this time, dogs have developed an innate and often uncannily accurate ability to recognize and adapt to humans' moods and interactions. Dogs know when we're sad. They know when we're annoyed. And they know how to get what they want: any dog can pull 'that look' to tug on the heart strings. (Even my cats – who spend most of the time roaming the village – let me know unequivocally when they want feeding or petting. I sometimes wonder who 'owns' whom.) This social intelligence allows dogs to integrate closely into our lives. In turn, we value this social intelligence (expressed as loyalty and so on) and, as a result, integrate dogs even more closely into our daily lives.

Healthcare professionals can use this intimate relationship to improve emotional, psychological and physical well-being – known as 'animal-facilitated therapy'. In addition, watching patients interact with animals can act as a window into thoughts, emotions and behaviour, which can guide care.[2]

A menagerie of therapeutic animals

For centuries, healers have used a menagerie of animals – including dogs, cats, guinea pigs, rabbits and horses – to bolster health and well-being. Handicapped people in Belgium helped care for farm animals in the ninth century. In the 1700s, the York Retreat – which was ahead of its time in treating people with mental illness – used rabbits, seagulls, hawks and other domestic animals, Sarah Matuszek remarks, to promote well-being and offer encouragement. Florence Nightingale suggested that a small pet 'is often an excellent companion' for sick people, especially those with chronic diseases.[2]

So why are animals therapeutic? In some cases, animals offer companionship; the care can help create a purpose in life and evoke pleasant memories, which help 'distract' people from a problem. And many people talk to their pets. Indeed, some people speak more openly to their pet than their spouse, probably because animals are, obviously, non-judgemental – and this helps get problems off the owner's chest.

Walking the dog can help prevent older people from becoming housebound, offer a sense of security and help exercise. Throwing an object for a dog to retrieve helps enhance coordination, builds upper body muscle strength and improves flexibility. Riding a horse improves posture, strength, balance and mobility even among patients with multiple sclerosis, cerebral palsy, spina bifida, autism and so on.[2]

Caring for and interacting with animals also alleviates stress and reduces blood pressure, heart rate and cholesterol levels. Even a fish tank in a dentist's waiting room is enough to reduce anxiety.[2] Petting animals can also give your immune system a boost. In one study, petting a dog for 18 minutes increased levels of IgA, an antibody in saliva, tears and other secretions that protects against bacteria, viruses and other pathogens. However, petting a stuffed dog or sitting on a sofa for the same time did not alter IgA production.[3] In other words, don't underestimate the strength of the bond between animals and humans or the benefits for your holistic health.

If you don't have a pet, speak to the Royal Society for the Prevention of Cruelty to Animals (RSPCA) or another animal charity to make sure that the animal you choose is right for you and that you will be able to look after it properly. If you have a suppressed immune system (you can catch some infections from animals) or an allergy it's worth checking with your doctor before you buy your pet.

A strong marriage

As a rule, married people live longer. (For the sake of brevity, 'married' encompasses other long-term, mutually supportive, cohabiting relationships with a 'significant other'.) For example, assuming that everything else remains the same, 90 per cent of married 48-year-old women will still be alive at 65 years of age compared to 80 per cent of those who never married. Men benefit even more: 90 per cent of married 48-year-old men will still be alive at 65 years of age, compared to just 60 per cent of life-long bachelors.[4]

Another study followed 4,802 40-year-old people for 22 years. Over this time, people who remained single were twice as likely to die prematurely than people who were consistently married, after allowing for personality and other risk factors. Divorced people were 64 per cent more likely to die prematurely.[5]

Not surprisingly, given the increased longevity, married people are less likely to suffer chronic illness, disability or physical problems than those who remain single. The difference is especially marked when behaviour or lifestyle makes a particular contribution to the illnesses.[4] For example, married patients were 2.5 times more likely to be alive 15 years after heart by-pass surgery than those who stayed single. Among people who said they were 'highly satisfied' with their marriage, men were almost three times, and women almost four times, more likely to be alive 15 years later. Indeed, a strong supportive marriage improved several factors linked to heart disease, such as abnormal increases in the size of the left ventricle (the heart's main blood-pumping chamber), blood pressure and chest pain.[6]

A surprising finding?

In some ways, the suggestion that a strong marriage and other social support networks help bolster your holistic health isn't surprising. Close family and friends and a strong marriage can give patients powerful 'reasons to live' as well as offering social, practical and emotional support to help you cope with stressful situations. Indeed, people with strong social connections show less marked changes in their blood pressure when they face high levels of negative emotions than those with fewer or weaker networks.[7] A spouse and friends can also give you a nudge to see a doctor when you feel unwell – which may be one reason why married people appear more likely to present with earlier stages of cancers.[8]

Furthermore, your partner's and family's practical and emotional support can be invaluable if you are trying to drink less alcohol, quit smoking, take more exercise, change your diet or take your medicines as prescribed. For example, your partner can help you adopt a healthy lifestyle, ignore bad moods triggered by the disease or lifestyle change, boost your motivation to stick to the plan when you feel like quitting and watch for side effects and harmful behaviours, such as offering a gentle reminder if you start eating unhealthy food regularly. Indeed, marriage's benefits in people who underwent by-pass surgery persisted for 15 years, reflecting the impact of lifestyle changes.[6]

Nevertheless, as mentioned when we looked at alcohol (page 58), deciding whether to tell your family, friends and colleagues that you are trying to change your lifestyle can sometimes be difficult. Some family and friends offer advice and support, especially if they have previously expressed concerns about your drinking, eating, smoking and so on. However, they might not be as understanding if you slip back: it is easy to underestimate how difficult changing your lifestyle can be. And some people may feel that you are challenging their lifestyle, and may prove hostile or condescending.

In other words, the quality of your social network matters as much as, if not more than, the quantity: you need to develop relationships that preserve or enhance your emotional well-being and bolster your ability to cope,[7] and disengage from those that are counterproductive. After all, social networks that encourage drug abuse or heavy drinking are hardly good for your health. In some cases, such as family or your work, you may not be able to remove yourself from the network. But you can probably find ways to limit their influence.

Similarly, a spouse's *support* – helping and reinforcing the partner's efforts to tackle unhealthy behaviours – improved the mental health of people after a heart attack or by-pass surgery. However, *control* – trying to persuade a partner to adopt healthy behaviours when he or she is unwilling or unable – reduced the likelihood that the patients would make the changes and undermined mental health.[9] Indeed, an experimental minor wound healed 40 per cent more slowly in those with 'hostile' marriages.[10] In other words, partners need to tread the fine line between 'nagging' and 'support'.

Marriage and adherence

Partners, family members and other carers can improve adherence (how well you follow your doctor's advice) by helping patients establish a routine for taking medicines. Some partners and family members write a list of the medicines the patient takes and when. You could give this list to an unfamiliar doctor (such as if you are on holiday), to accident and emergency staff and to pharmacists if you are buying medication. Some medicines can interact with other drugs, either causing side effects or undermining effectiveness.

Sex life and chronic diseases

A sex life that is right for you and your partner helps build and maintain relationships. However, stress, depression, anxiety and several physical conditions (e.g. diabetes and cardiovascular disease) can cause impotence or undermine your sex drive. A stoma bag or a skin disease, for instance, can be off-putting for both partners. Indeed, Russell notes, the impact on sex life 'is often the most distressing aspect of a chronic illness'. Yet 'fear of embarrassment' means that many doctors don't ask about their patients' sex lives.

In some cases – such as asthma or angina – physical activity can trigger an attack. Try talking to a counsellor or ask your doctor, nurse or patient group what may help: this may include not having sex after a heavy meal, not drinking too much alcohol, creating a relaxing atmosphere and getting into a comfortable position. Your partner may take a more active role. Remember to keep your angina spray, asthma inhaler or any other medications you need by the bed. A romantic mood and tackling any issues can help reinvigorate a sex life that stalls in the wake of a serious disease.

In other cases, some drugs (including some antidepressants, beta-blockers and calcium antagonists) or diseases (e.g. diabetes, atherosclerosis and depression) can affect your sex drive or cause impotence. Speak to your GP if you think a medicine or a poorly controlled ailment could cause your impotence or reduced sex drive. Switching treatment may resolve the problem. In addition, GPs and some pharmacists can offer Viagra (sildenafil) and a growing range of other effective treatments for male impotence (properly called erectile dysfunction). But never buy any drug over the internet, unless you are sure the online pharmacy is reputable.

Look after yourself

Caring for a person with a serious disease can be physically demanding, emotionally draining and highly disruptive. So, to look after your partner you need to look after yourself.

Try to sleep or unwind while your partner is resting and get a good night's sleep – the following box offers some tips that may help patients as well as carers. You should follow any advice offered by the specialist, GP or nurse about the patient's activity. You might feel you want to do more than this. However, your good intentions could hinder recovery and place an unnecessary burden on your shoulders. If your partner is recovering from a serious operation or illness, think about limiting the number of visitors you have and how long they stay. Finally, make sure you have time to yourself.

You might need to be honest with yourself. A serious disease can leave your partner mentally and emotionally devastated. He or she may live overshadowed by stress and practical problems, be afraid of dying, and feel upset at not being able to take part in previously enjoyed activities. Not surprisingly, people with a serious disease might feel depressed, angry, guilty and bad-tempered, which can place a strain on your relationships.

On the other hand, partners of people with serious diseases often feel angry, guilty and resentful. And other family members may

Tips for a good night's sleep

You can take several steps to help you sleep better without resorting to sleeping pills:

- Wind down or relax at the end of the day: do not go to bed while your mind is racing or pondering problems.
- Try not to take your troubles to bed with you. Brooding on problems makes them seem worse, exacerbates stress, keeps you awake and, because you're tired in the morning, means you are less able to deal with your difficulties. Try to avoid heavy discussions before bed.
- Do not worry about anything you have forgotten to do. Get up and jot it down (keep a notepad by the bed if you find you do this commonly). This should help you forget about the problem until the morning.
- Go to bed at the same time each night and set your alarm for the same time each morning, even at the weekends. This helps re-establish a regular sleep pattern.
- Avoid naps during the day.
- Avoid stimulants, such as caffeine and nicotine, for several hours before bed. Try hot milk or milky drinks instead.
- Do not drink too much fluid (even if non-alcoholic) just before bed as this can mean regular trips to the bathroom.
- Avoid alcohol. A nightcap can help you fall asleep, but as blood levels fall sleep becomes more fragmented and lighter. Therefore, you may wake repeatedly in the latter part of the night.
- Do not eat a heavy meal before bedtime.
- Although regular exercise helps you sleep, exercising just before bed can disrupt sleep.
- Use the bed for sex and sleep only. Do not work or watch TV.
- Make the bed and bedroom as comfortable as possible. Invest in a comfortable mattress, with enough bedclothes, and make sure the room is not too hot, too cold or too bright.
- If you cannot sleep, get up and do something else. Watch the TV or read – nothing too stimulating – until you feel tired. Lying there worrying about not sleeping just keeps you awake.

feel they don't receive sufficient attention. Do not bottle these feelings up: as we have already seen, conflict between people and in marriages can undermine health and well-being. Indeed, concealing or repressing your emotional pain and stress (or, indeed, a patient bottling things up) can erode closeness in relationships. So, think and talk about your feelings with your partner, friends and family or even a counsellor. Carers Direct is a national information, advice and support service for carers in England (<www.nhs.uk/carersdirect>; 0808 802 0202).

Employment

Many of us count the days until Friday night – or the years until retirement. Yet employment (even if it's unpaid) can help recovery from a serious illness and often bolsters health and well-being. As we've seen, unemployment can increase the risk of developing numerous mental and physical diseases. And returning to work after a serious disease reduces the risk of depression – partly because it is a sign that you're on the road to recovery.

Yet many people who could work (even part-time and in voluntary roles) do not. (I should stress that I do not support 'forcing' people who are sick or disabled back to work by attacking benefits. However, helping people back into employment can aid rehabilitation and help get life back to normal.) For example, according to the British Heart Foundation, around a third of people who suffer a heart attack in the UK are under 65 years of age. Two-thirds of these are in employment when they suffer their heart attack, but up to half never return to work. Many probably could have worked, although they may need several months to recover.

You, your employer and your doctor need to strike a delicate balance. The longer you wait, the less likely you are to return to work. However, some symptoms – such as chest pain and breathlessness – may reduce the chance of returning to work or at least delay your return. Depressed patients, not surprisingly, are less likely than more optimistic people to return to work.

Furthermore, you are less likely to return if you believe that stress at work caused or made an important contribution to your illness. Other people believe that the illness is a warning that they are 'worn out' and need to 'take things easy' – which may mean giving up their job. In addition, people who believe that their ailment will have a long-term impact on their health are much less likely to return to work than those who see the illness as a 'short-term' problem.

So, ask your doctor's advice about whether and when you can return to work, and whether your job contributed to your ailment. Occasionally, an occupational therapist may need to assess the workplace and work with you to develop a plan that minimizes, for example, physical strain, fatigue and the effect of poor concentration. You may need to ease yourself back gently into the 'daily grind' – such as beginning with alternate half-days at work and light or less challenging duties rather than throwing yourself immediately back into the fray – and gradually build up over several weeks.

The business of spirituality

Some companies, Sheldrake comments, now try to integrate spirituality into the workplace. This can range from starting the day with tai chi or offering meditation at lunch-time to formulating a ethical value system to underpin the business. This approach engenders a sense of meaning and purpose that goes beyond production alone. Advocates claim that organizations that integrate spirituality into their business tend to attract the best staff and improve motivation and company performance.

Stress on the job

While employment can be a source of satisfaction and fulfilment, your job can also be a major cause of stress – and trigger ill health – if, for example, you do not get on with your colleagues, you feel underappreciated and over-worked, or your pay cheque leaves you short each month. Indeed, while executive stress remains almost a badge of honour in some companies, senior managers control their working life much more than their subordinates. An executive's workload tends to be more varied and interesting than those lower down the corporate ladder – and boredom drives stress. Moreover, seniority brings financial rewards that allow executives to make the most of their leisure time – an important stress defence.

As a rule, a company's most stressed-out employees tend to be those who work long hours in repetitive jobs with little control for relatively low pay: production-line workers, checkout assistants, call-centre staff and so on. For example:

- One analysis looked at 38 studies evaluating the link between stress and mental disorders, such as anxiety, depression and suicide. People with limited opportunities to take decisions at work were 21 per cent more likely to develop a mental health problem than those with more control. Those who experienced poor relationships at work were 32 per cent more likely to develop mental health problems.[11]
- People who felt there was a marked discrepancy between the effort they put in and the reward they received were 84 per cent more likely to develop mental health issues.[11]
- Repeated job strain more than doubled (119 per cent increase) the risk of depression over a decade. Repeated low social support at work increased the risk of depression by 61 per cent.[12]

A skills audit

Suffering from a serious disease may change many areas of your life. Some changes may arise from limitations imposed by the illness. In other cases, a chronic disease may lead you to re-evaluate your priorities in life generally as well as in your job.

A skills audit (Table 6.1) can help you decide on the most appropriate career change – or, if you already have a goal in mind, how you can attain your ambition. This means looking critically, but realistically, at your current situation. You can also use this approach when writing a CV or if you face particular problems at work – such as less experienced people being promoted over you because they offer specific skills.

Make a list of all the jobs you have held. Against each one, try to list between three and six things you have learnt – both specific skills and personally. Then try to list between three and six ways in which you made a difference. Remember, even the worst job – and I speak from bitter experience – adds to your skill set and teaches you something.

Next, decide your goal. Perhaps you already know, broadly, what you want to do. Often the skills audit will clarify the sort of job that

Teaching old dogs new tricks

It's never too late to set new goals or learn new skills. The psychologist Carl Jung noted in the 1930s that many people found their life devoid of meaning or purpose when they grew older. Today, older people can use the opportunity to develop interests or rediscover a hobby for which they never had time when they needed to earn a living and bring up a family. They may become more actively involved in the church or another voluntary organization. They may take a course at the Open University. Not being tied down to a routine imposed by earning a living offers something of a blank canvas.

Table 6.1 Essential elements of a skills audit

- Educational qualifications
- Professional qualifications – formal and informal (e.g. training courses)
- Your interests at work – what interests you about your job, even if it is just meeting people
- The practical skills you use at work
- Your knowledge at work – which may be more than you currently use
- What do you dislike about your job? What makes you feel frustrated?
- Your interests outside work
- Your skills outside work
- Your knowledge outside work
- What do you dislike about life outside work? What makes you feel frustrated?
- Any awards you've won – even employee of the month
- Your job history, what you've learnt and your successes
- Your roles outside work – church, Scouts, a football team

will suit you, especially if you compare what you like about your job and what you dislike. There may well be a skills gap that hinders your ability to realize your ambitions or attain your potential in your current job. You can ask the Open University, your human relations manager, adult learning centre and so on whether any course will fill the gap.

Objectively SMART

The audit should reveal the skills you need. Convert each skill shortage into a goal that is SMART: Specific, Measurable, Attainable, Relevant and Time-framed. In some cases, you may have to break larger goals into smaller objectives. Ideally, these should be steps that you can take regularly – each week, even each day – and that will take you closer. Set a 'deadline' – then add 10 per cent or 20 per cent to your estimate. Most people underestimate how long a change will take. You may also want to set a budget. Again, add 10–20 per cent to ensure that you have enough.

Each change should be attainable and relevant to your ultimate objective. Failing to meet your expectations or going off along an irrelevant by-way can waste time and money as well as undermine your confidence. Then review your progress regularly. This proactive approach can help you find the rewarding work that helps – rather than hinders – your holistic health.

7

Resilience and the road to recovery

Healthy people often don't realize just how stressful suffering from a serious disease can prove. Indeed, post-traumatic stress disorder (PTSD) can follow in the wake of a serious disease, operation or other adversity. Patients with PTSD often report flashbacks that emerge 'out of the blue' and vivid dreams and nightmares. They also typically avoid places and people that evoke memories of the trauma, refuse to speak about their experiences and feel constantly on guard or emotionally numb.

PTSD is common after the horrors of sexual assault, physical attack or military combat: UK reservists deployed to Iraq in 2003 were around 2.4 times more likely to develop PTSD during the next five years than those who remained at home.[1] However, PTSD can also follow physical or mental illness – such as cancer, HIV infection or a mental breakdown. Indeed, around a quarter of people who suffer acute coronary syndrome (heart attacks and a related condition called unstable angina) develop PTSD.[2] See your doctor if you feel that you may have PTSD, which blights lives, places a considerable strain on relationships and increases the risk of drug and alcohol abuse.

On the other hand, some people emerge from, or live with, very serious physical or mental illnesses, injury or trauma apparently unscathed. Rather than developing PTSD or descending into despair and depression, they use adversity, illness and trauma as a springboard to personal and spiritual growth. After all, adversity challenges your assumptions and forces you to examine your core beliefs. As such, adversity offers the opportunity and motivation to improve relationships, recognize new possibilities, and increase appreciation for your blessings and aid spiritual development.

Indeed, the 'positive psychology' movement shifts the focus from repairing damage caused by life's problems to identifying and building on each person's strengths and virtues. Positive psychology buffers us against adversity and protects from psychological issues once problems emerge.[3] So, how can you move along the road to recovery? How can you bolster your resilience? And how can you develop the mind set that allows you to focus on problems while regulating your emotional distress?

Well on the road to recovery

Based on his experiences in the trenches of the First World War, Dr Charles Wilson (later Baron Moran) argued in *The Anatomy of Courage* that people start with different amounts of courage – one facet of resilience. Problems deplete your stores of courage – the terror of the Passchendaele trenches more rapidly than the unreasonable demands of a tyrannical boss. Rest and recuperation help restore some of your resources. However, eventually your reserves of courage might run out.

Courage means different things to different people at different times in their lives. The courage an infantry solider needs to patrol in a hostile country is different from the courage a severely depressed person needs to go to work or an alcoholic needs to stop drinking. But all require courage. Some people have enough courage and other inner resources to tough things out on their own. However, most of us need help along the road to recovery.

Against this background, researchers looked at 97 studies and identified five 'recovery processes' among people with mental health problems (which can also apply to many other chronic diseases):

- connectedness
- hope and optimism
- a sense of identity
- finding meaning in life
- empowerment.[4]

We've discussed several of these processes over the course of the book. For example:

- We've seen that people in stable, supportive relationships – exemplified by good marriages (page 90) – tend to develop positive coping strategies.
- In Chapter 3, we saw that religion and some spiritual movements

offer social networks and support – connectedness – that help you along the road to recovery.

- Religion and spirituality can help you understand the meaning of life and develop a sense of identity (Chapter 3).
- As you learn that you can cope with your problems, you'll develop a sense of empowerment.

So, in this section, we'll focus on why doing your best to remain optimistic helps bolster holistic health.

Hope and optimism

Hope, optimism and positive emotions generally may help restore your mental and physical resources, build long-lasting social resources and enhance well-being despite intense stress. In addition, positive emotions increase your flexibility of thinking and enhance problem-solving.[5] And remember that emotions are contagious. If you keep optimistic, it's more likely that the people around you will remain optimistic, creating a virtuous cycle.

For example, a study of women with early breast cancer found that those who felt helpless, hopeless and depressed were 55 per cent more likely to die over the next five years than those with a more positive outlook. Another study included women with advanced breast cancer that had spread to other parts of their body (metastasis). Women who minimized the malignancy's impact on their social, work and family lives survived for around five months longer than those who couldn't adapt as well (on average, about 29 and 24 months respectively).[6] The first step to developing a positive outlook is to take humour seriously.

Taking laughter seriously

Occasionally, people die laughing. As mentioned earlier (page 48), strong emotions, even when positive, can increase the risk of suffering a heart attack. More commonly, however, laughter is therapeutic. As the great seventeenth-century English physician Thomas Sydenham remarked: 'The arrival of a single clown has a more healthful impact on the health of a village than that of twenty asses laden with medications.'

Psychoanalysts who follow the teachings of Sigmund Freud believe humour 'distances' us from the problem, places issues in perspective, reframes the problem and minimizes distress.[7] In other words, laughter helps create a constructive mental outlook that aids problem-solving.[8] In addition, humour counters stress, depression, insomnia and loneliness, and enhances self-esteem, hope, mood, energy and vigour.[7, 9] And laughter releases the tension generated by fear and anger. Similarly, tears discharge the tension that accompanies sadness.

Laughter and tears produce a range of biological benefits, including countering overactivity of the sympathetic nervous system (page 23). Initially, laughter and tears increase levels of adrenaline and noradrenaline in the blood, which, in turn, speeds heart rate and elevates blood pressure – some hallmarks of sympathetic nervous activity. A relaxation phase, controlled by the parasympathetic nervous system, follows – which is why you may feel 'pleasantly drained' after laughing or crying.[8]

Laughter's biological benefits

Laughter produces a range of biological benefits including:

- exercising and relaxing muscles;
- improving respiration, especially by promoting deep breathing (page 23);
- stimulating blood circulation;
- decreasing levels of stress hormones;
- bolstering immune defences;
- increasing the pain threshold and tolerance;
- enhancing mental functioning, including memory, creative thinking and problem-solving.

Laughter and tears also reduce the 'social and emotional distance between people', which, in turn, helps generate compassion, encourages human contact and resolves interpersonal conflicts.[8] Indeed, laughter possibly evolved as a signal of safety and security to other people.[7] In other words, laughter and tears help build the social structures, cohesiveness and relationships that protect against stress, and help us cope with the challenges associated with living with a chronic disease (Chapter 6).[9]

Indeed, the benefits are so marked that some hospitals and hospices run laughter and humour sessions – including visits from clowns – teach laughter meditation or run laughter clubs.[7] Another way is to curl up with a comedy DVD, CD or book. You may have the last laugh over your disease.

Adverse coping

In contrast, psychologists identified several traits that undermine resilience and exacerbate psychological distress:[5]

- over-reacting to minor hassles, problems and stress;
- regarding negative events as especially harmful;
- experiencing a greater number of negative events – the more problems you have, the more your resources are depleted;
- allowing spill-over from negative mood generally – people with depression or a low mood are less able to cope and remain optimistic;
- being unable to adjust to recurring problems.

Several adverse coping strategies alleviate the anxiety triggered by a disease, trauma or adversity by 'distorting' reality or altering self-perception. In some cases and for a short time these can tide you over a rough patch and allow you to tackle your immediate issues. However, allowing an adverse coping strategy to become entrenched can leave you unable to deal with your problems.

Repression and denial

As we saw with PTSD, repression is a powerful defence: we banish discomforting, unpleasant thoughts or guilty memories from the conscious mind. However, these thoughts lurk in the subconscious and can re-emerge – sometimes as a flashback, but in a distorted, almost unrecognizable form – triggering stress and undermining our ability to cope. In some cases, people may experience flashbacks. In other cases, psychoanalysts may need to uncover forgotten memories that are causing stress.

Denial is similar to repression but focuses on current challenges rather than the past. Denial allows us to avoid accepting the reality of our situation – even when faced with overwhelming evidence. For example, many drug addicts, gamblers and alcoholics minimize or deny the harm that they are doing to themselves and others. Alcoholics Anonymous and other rehabilitation programmes succeed partly because they help people face their addiction and deal with its consequences.

Similarly, terminally ill people (page 40) or those who have contracted a chronic infection (such as HIV or hepatitis C virus) may deny the truth until they can muster the emotional, psychological and practical resources to face reality. However, denial may mean that people do not get the treatment they need or change a harmful lifestyle. So, you may need to gently and sympathetically encourage the person to seek help.

Aggression and anger

Aggression and anger are common reactions when you learn you have a serious disease or face the problems of living with that condition. Anger can prove a valuable safety valve. My father's DIY exploits regularly expanded my childhood lexicon of expletives. Hitting the nail on his thumb, rather the nail in the wall, would unleash an angry stream of swear words. Despite my mother's objections, it made him feel better. And as we've seen (page 40) anger is a common and natural response to life-changing news.

However, excessive, protracted aggression and anger can mean you do not address the problem. And when directed against a person or object, anger and aggression can frighten those around you and may even lead to legal complications. Try to accept your anger and channel your emotions more productively. You might find that talking to a counsellor or your religious adviser can help you understand why you react with anger when faced with your problems and develop a more effective coping mechanism.

Withdrawal

Withdrawal is another common response to stress and adversity. Retreating into a mental shell can offer a strategic withdrawal allowing us the time and space to re-evaluate our lives, priorities and problems. However, some people narrow their horizons until their lives are within limits they think they can control, which may be very limited indeed. Taken to extremes, withdrawal encourages apathy, depression and isolation from the social networks that support holistic health.

Understanding your problems

Existing and new problems can hinder your progress along the road to recovery – and trigger denial, withdrawal, anger and so on. However, sometimes even identifying your problem can pose a challenge, especially if you're in denial. In other cases, you may not be able to work out whether it's the disease (e.g. pain or another symptom) or the impact it has on your life (such as stopping a valued activity) that is more distressing. And problems elsewhere in your life can make you feel even more unwell and may encourage you to re-evaluate your mental and spiritual priorities. So, on a blank piece of paper, try to answer the following questions:

- *What is the problem?* Try to state the problem as a clear simple sentence. 'The pressure at work is making me unwell.' 'My smoking means I can't exercise.' 'I can't control my drinking.' If you cannot state the problem in a single sentence, you may have more than one issue. Try breaking the problem down. You can also home in on the fundamentals by considering what the problem is not, or when it arises: 'I do not drink unless I have to make a presentation at work.'
- *Who contributes to the problem?* List everyone who influences the problem or your response. Then consider who makes matters worse and who helps. Now ask yourself: 'What have I contributed?' Be honest. Most of us lay the blame at someone else's feet – so-called transference. On the other hand, try not to blame yourself for events outside your control or for the actions of others.
- *Where and when does the problem occur?* At home? At work? Many smokers and people who drink or eat excessively respond to environmental and emotional cues (page 51). Understanding where a problem occurs can help uncover why it arises. As mentioned before, keeping a diary can reveal patterns and triggers. For example, some women feel depressed or suffer a migraine just before their period. Other people may drink when visiting relatives who base their social life around alcohol.

Your answers may reveal patterns and suggest possible solutions. For instance, assertiveness training may help if you drink to bolster your self-confidence. Relaxation therapy may help if you smoke because you are stressed. Blocking time in your diary or adding exercise to your everyday activities (page 49) may help if you cannot find the time to exercise. A skills audit (page 97) can help you address many problems at work.

Boosting resilience

Positive coping strategies help bolster your resilience in particular and your holistic health more generally. Essentially, resilient people cope with stress, risk and adversity better than you might expect given the problems they face.[5] Researchers identified some core 'protective factors' (many of which will, by now, seem familiar) that seem to contribute to resilience. They broadly separate into:

- *Individual attributes, such as an easy-going temperament and well-developed abilities to control our behaviour* Partly, our level of resilience is genetic. (Remember the idea that we're all born with a certain reserve of courage – page 101.) Partly, our resilience depends on our upbringing. And partly our experiences forge resilience as we face the problems life throws up.
- *Strong, close relationships* These are characterized by trust, warmth and cohesion in families and with other people.
- *External support* This may be in our neighbourhood, schools, churches and so on.[5]

Are you ego-resilient or brittle?

Psychologists differentiate 'ego-resilient' and 'ego-brittle' children. Ego-resilient children tend to be 'confident, perceptive, insightful' and 'form warm and open' relationships; they can overcome, navigate and recover from adversity. 'Ego-brittle' children, in contrast, tend to experience more behavioural problems, depression and drug use during adolescence. And these differences extend into adulthood. In one study, people with high ego resilience were less likely to suffer depression after the attacks in the USA on September 11, 2001.[5]

Locus of control

These three mutually reinforcing strands mean that resilient people tend to feel in control of events. Psychologists describe the extent to which you feel you control your life as your 'locus of control'. If you have a strong external locus of control, you see yourself as having little influence over your life. You feel that events control you; you do not control events. A strong internal locus of control means that you tend to see yourself as in charge of your life. People with a strong internal locus are, generally, less likely to be stressed out than those with an external locus of control. Indeed, INTERHEART (page 46) found that a high internal locus of control reduced the risk that people would suffer their first heart attack by 32 per cent.[10]

On the other hand, feeling helpless in one part of your life can spill over into other areas. For example, if you feel disempowered – that events and circumstances are beyond your control – or you feel that your life 'is over' because of, for example, breathing problems or heart disease, you may be less able to make the changes needed to stop smoking or start drinking safely or eating healthily.

You can enhance your internal locus of control by actively taking steps to improve your holistic health and well-being. Being a passive recipient of health care, just popping the pills, means control lies 'externally' with your doctor. In contrast, reading about and trying to understand your disease as well as following your doctor's advice and proactively addressing an unhealthy lifestyle enhances your internal locus of control. As you address your problems, as you take control of your health, as you reduce your risk factors, you will feel more and more confident. This, in turn, bolsters your internal locus of control and boosts your resilience.

Summing up

The American Psychological Association proposed ten ways that help build resilience – which will not come as a surprise after reading this book. (I've slightly adapted these in line with the rest of the book. You can find the original here: <www.apa.org/helpcenter/road-resilience.aspx>.) Indeed, these ten points summarize the key ways to bolster your holistic health.

Make connections and relations

Develop a social network by establishing supportive relationships with family, friends, voluntary and other groups, religious organizations and charities. Many people find that helping others benefits them in times of difficulty. Do not be afraid to express your emotions. Discuss your problems and accept help and support from other people.

Acknowledge that you can overcome your problems

Your problems are not insurmountable. You cannot alter events in the past and if, for example, you face a terminal illness, you may not be able to change the future. So, try to accept your emotional and physical pain, your illness or your problems. Remember, even if you can't change your circumstances, you can alter your reaction.

Accept that everything changes

The Greek philosopher Heraclitus famously commented, about 2,500 years ago, 'Everything changes, nothing stays still . . . You cannot step into the same stream twice.' You may need to accept that circumstances mean you can no longer attain a once-treasured ambition. You may need to rethink your goals and re-evaluate your ambitions.

On the other hand, there may be nothing you can do if, for example, you develop a life-threatening illness. So, accept that some circumstances cannot be changed. Even for atheists, Reinhold Niebuhr's 'Serenity Prayer' eloquently sums up this approach:

God, grant me the serenity to accept the things I cannot change,
Courage to change the things I can,
And the wisdom to know the difference.

Develop and move towards realistic goals

As we suggested in the skills audit (page 97), try to take small steps – every day if you can, and even if it is a relatively minor advance – that take you closer to your goal. Remember to break large goals into smaller steps and make each objective SMART (page 99).

Do not be passive

Withdrawing excessively or hoping your problems will sort themselves out (a type of denial) are common adverse coping strategies (page 104). You need to identify your problems and take action. Being proactive helps engender an internal locus of control.

Make the most of the problem

As we have seen, a problem can be part of your voyage of self-discovery. Many people experience 'post-traumatic growth' in their relationships, with a sense of inner strength, self-worth, spirituality and a heightened appreciation for life.

Keep your problems in perspective

Try to take a broader view by – for example – focusing on other parts of your life. Try to count your blessings; some people even make a list. Try to avoid making mountains out of molehills. You could ask yourself whether the problem will still be an issue in six months' or a year's time. Humour (page 102), literature and the other arts, visiting museums, walking in nature (page 49) can help create and maintain a sense of perspective.

Look after yourself

What do you need to do to help yourself cope? Find the time to take part in activities that you enjoy. Relax and exercise regularly. You may need to find the time to take a more active approach to relaxation (page 80).

Find other ways to bolster your inner resources

You could keep a diary (page 10), meditate or invest more time in your spiritual practices.

Stay positive and nurture hope and optimism

Develop confidence in your ability to solve problems and trust your instincts. An active approach to tackling problems can help. Success breeds success. Moving towards your goal boosts your confidence. Don't forget about the healing power of humour.

We have already seen that optimism and hope aid recovery. Try focusing on your goals, rather than worrying about your anxieties or ruminating on your current problems. But do not let this distract you from taking action to deal with your problems.

I will leave the last word to William Osler – one of the greatest clinicians in the eighteenth and early nineteenth centuries. Osler reported the case of a patient bedridden with metastatic breast cancer. The malignancy had spread to her spine, other breast and right eye. Two years later, Osler reported, 'She drove a mile and a half to the station to meet me and drove me to the station on my return.' Osler said the case – and others like it – 'are among the most remarkable' in medicine. And the case illustrates the main message of this book: 'no condition, however desperate, is quite hopeless'.[11]

Useful addresses

**Action on Smoking and Health
(ASH)**
Sixth Floor, Suites 59–63
New House, 67–68 Hatton Garden
London EC1N 8JY
Tel.: 020 7404 0242
Website: www.ash.org.uk

Alcohol Concern
Suite B5, West Wing
New City Cloisters
196 Old Street
London EC1V 9FR
Tel.: 020 7566 9800
Website: www.alcoholconcern.org.uk

**British Association for
Counselling and Psychotherapy**
BACP House
15 St John's Business Park
Lutterworth
Leics LE17 4HB
Tel.: 01455 883300
Website: www.bacp.co.uk

**British Association of Medical
Hypnosis**
45 Hyde Park Square
London W2 2JY
Website: www.bamh.org.uk

British Dietetic Association
Fifth Floor, Charles House
148/9 Great Charles Street
Queensway
Birmingham B3 3HT
Tel.: 0121 200 8080
Website: www.bda.uk.com/index.html

British Heart Foundation
Greater London House
180 Hampstead Road
London NW1 7AW
Tel.: 0300 330 3311 (helpline)
Website: www.bhf.org.uk

British Liver Trust
2 Southampton Road
Ringwood
Hants BH24 1HY
Tel.: 0800 652 7330 (helpline)
Website: www.britishlivertrust.org.uk

British Wheel of Yoga
25 Jermyn Street
Sleaford
Lincs NG34 7RU
Tel.: 01529 306851
Website: www.bwy.org.uk

Cancer Research UK
Angel Building
407 St John Street
London EC1V 4AD
Tel.: 0808 800 4040 (helpline)
Website: www.cancerresearchuk.org

Child Bereavement Trust
Clare Charity Centre
Wycombe Road
Saunderton
Bucks HP14 4BF
Tel.: 01494 568900
Website: www.childbereavement.
org.uk

Complementary and Natural
Healthcare Council
83 Victoria Street
London SW1H 0HW
Tel.: 020 3178 2199
Website: www.cnhc.org.uk

Cruse Bereavement Care
PO Box 800
Richmond
Surrey TW9 1RG
Tel.: 020 8939 9530
Helpline: 0844 477 9400
Website: www.cruse.org.uk

Diabetes UK
Macleod House
10 Parkway
London NW1 7AA
Tel.: 020 7424 1000
Careline: 0845 120 2960
Website: www.diabetes.org.uk

General Regulatory Council for
Complementary Therapies
Box 437, Office 6
Slington House
Rankine Road
Basingstoke RG24 8PH
Tel.: 0870 3144031
Website: www.grcct.org

Health and Care Professionals
Council
Park House
184 Kennington Park Road
London SE11 4BU
Tel.: 020 7820 9684
Website: www.hpc-uk.org

Institute for Complementary and
Natural Medicine (and British
Register of Complementary
Practitioners)
Can Mezzanine
32–36 Loman Street
London SE1 0EH
Tel.: 020 7922 7980
Website: www.icnm.org.uk

Macmillan Cancer Support
89 Albert Embankment
London SE1 7UQ
Tel.: 0808 808 00 00 (helpline)
Website: www.macmillan.org.uk

National Organisation for Foetal
Alcohol Syndrome (NOFAS-UK)
165 Beaufort Park
London NW11 6DA
Helpline: 020 8458 5951
Website: www.nofas-uk.org

National Osteoporosis Society
Camerton
Bath BA2 0PJ
Tel.: 0845 450 0230 (helpline)
Website: www.nos.org.uk

Royal Society for the Prevention
of Cruelty to Animals (RSPCA)
Wilberforce Way
Southwater
Horsham
West Sussex RH13 9RS
Tel.: 0300 1234 999 (helpline)
Website: www.rspca.org.uk

Stroke Association
Stroke House
240 City Road
London EC1V 2PR
Tel.: 020 7566 0300
Helpline: 0303 303 3100
Website: www.stroke.org.uk

The Tai Chi Union for Great
Britain
1 Littlemill Drive
Glasgow G53 7GF
Website: www.taichiunion.com

References

Introduction

1 Papac, R.J. Spontaneous regression of cancer. *Cancer Treatment Reviews* 1996; **22**: 395–423.

2 Maggiore, R.J., Gross, C.P., Togawa, K. et al. Use of complementary medications among older adults with cancer. *Cancer* 2012; **118**: 4815–23.

3 Hajdu, S.I. A note from history: landmarks in history of cancer, part 4. *Cancer* 2012; **118**: 4914–28.

4 Foukakis, T., Fornander, T., Lekberg, T., Hellborg, H., Adolfsson, J. and Bergh, J. Age-specific trends of survival in metastatic breast cancer: 26 years longitudinal data from a population-based cancer registry in Stockholm, Sweden. *Breast Cancer Research and Treatment* 2011; **130**: 553–60.

5 *A Century of Change: Trends in UK Statistics since 1900*. House of Commons Library Research Paper 99/111, 21 December 1999; <www.parliament.uk/commons/lib/research/rp99/rp99-111.pdf>.

6 Brown, K. 'That's funny!': the discovery and development of penicillin. *Microbiology Today* 2009; **36** (1): 12–15.

7 Breo, D.L. The US race to 'cure' AIDS – at '4' on a scale of 10, says Dr Fauci. *JAMA: The Journal of the American Medical Association* 1993; **269**: 2898–900.

8 *Mortality Statistics: Deaths registered in 2008. Review of the National Statistician on deaths in England and Wales, 2008*. London: Office of National Statistics, 2009; <www.statistics.gov.uk/downloads/theme_health/DR2008/DR_08.pdf>.

9 Vallance, A.K. Something out of nothing: the placebo effect. *Advances in Psychiatric Treatment* 2006; **12**: 287–96.

10 Dugan, D.O. Laughter and tears: best medicine for stress. *Nursing Forum* 1989; **24**: 18–26.

11 Bond, C., Blenkinsopp, A. and Raynor, D.K. Prescribing and partnership with patients. *British Journal of Clinical Pharmacology* 2012; **74**: 581–8.

1 The limitations of modern medicine

1 Tikkinen, K.A.O., Leinonen, J.S., Guyatt, G.H., Ebrahim, S. and Järvinen, T.L.N. What is a disease? Perspectives of the public, health professionals and legislators. *BMJ Open* 2012; **2**: e001632.

2 Boehm, J.K., Peterson, C., Kivimaki, M. and Kubzansky, L.D. Heart health when life is satisfying: evidence from the Whitehall II cohort study. *European Heart Journal* 2011; **32**: 2672–7.

3 Mueller, P.S., Plevak, D.J. and Rummans, T.A. Religious involvement, spirituality, and medicine: implications for clinical practice. *Mayo Clinic Proceedings* 2001; **76**: 1225–35.

4 Gramenzi, A., Caputo, F., Biselli, M. et al. Review article: alcoholic liver disease – pathophysiological aspects and risk factors. *Alimentary Pharmacology & Therapeutics* 2006; **24**: 1151–61.

5 Vickers, A.J., Cronin, A.M., Maschino, A.C. et al. Acupuncture for chronic pain: individual patient data meta-analysis. *Archives of Internal Medicine* 2012; **172**: 1444–53.

6 Pergolizzi, J., Boger, R.H., Budd, K. et al. Opioids and the management of chronic severe pain in the elderly: consensus statement of an International Expert Panel with focus on the six clinically most often used World Health Organization Step III opioids (buprenorphine, fentanyl, hydromorphone, methadone, morphine, oxycodone). *Pain Practice: The Official Journal of World Institute of Pain* 2008; **8**: 287–313.

7 Kalager, M., Adami, H.-O., Bretthauer, M. and Tamimi, R.M. Overdiagnosis of invasive breast cancer due to mammography screening: results from the Norwegian screening program. *Annals of Internal Medicine* 2012; **156**: 491–9.

8 Moynihan, R., Doust, J. and Henry, D. Preventing overdiagnosis: how to stop harming the healthy. *British Medical Journal* 2012; **344**: e3502.

9 Riley, T.R., III, and Bhatti, A.M. Preventive strategies in chronic liver disease: part I. Alcohol, vaccines, toxic medications and supplements, diet and exercise. *American Family Physician* 2001; **64**: 1555–60.

10 Pirmohamed, M., James, S., Meakin, S. et al. Adverse drug reactions as cause of admission to hospital: prospective analysis of 18 820 patients. *British Medical Journal* 2004; **329**: 15–19.

11 Ernst, E. Risks of herbal medicinal products. *Pharmacoepidemiology and Drug Safety* 2004; **13**: 767–71.

12 Hajdu, S.I. A note from history: landmarks in history of cancer, part 4. *Cancer* 2012; **118**: 4914–28.

13 Al-Arouj, M., Bouguerra, R., Buse, J. et al. Recommendations for management of diabetes during Ramadan. *Diabetes Care* 2005; **28**: 2305–11.

14 Sloman, R., Rosen, G., Rom, M. and Shir, Y. Nurses' assessment of pain in surgical patients. *Journal of Advanced Nursing* 2005; **52**: 125–32.

15 Rajasagaram, U., Taylor, D.M., Braitberg, G., Pearsell, J.P. and Capp, B.A. Paediatric pain assessment: differences between triage nurse, child and parent. *Journal of Paediatrics and Child Health* 2009; **45**: 199–203.

16 Citrome, L. Compelling or irrelevant? How using number needed to treat can help decide. *Acta Psychiatrica Scandinavica* 2008; **117**: 412–19.

17 Gadsby, R., Galloway, M., Barker, P. and Sinclair, A. Prescribed medicines for elderly frail people with diabetes resident in nursing homes – issues of polypharmacy and medication costs. *Diabetic Medicine* 2012; **29**: 136–9.

18 Banerjee, A., Mbamalu, D., Ebrahimi, S., Khan, A.A. and Chan, T.F. The prevalence of polypharmacy in elderly attenders to an emergency department – a problem with a need for an effective solution. *International Journal of Emergency Medicine* 2011; **4**: 22.

19 Osterberg, L. and Blaschke, T. Adherence to medication. *The New England Journal of Medicine* 2005; **353**: 487–97.
20 Yang, Y., Thumula, V., Pace, P.F., Banahan, B.F., III, Wilkin, N.E. and Lobb, W.B. Predictors of medication nonadherence among patients with diabetes in Medicare Part D programs: a retrospective cohort study. *Clinical Therapeutics* 2009; **31**: 2178–88; discussion 2150–1.
21 Rodriguez, L.A., Cea-Soriano, L., Martin-Merino, E. and Johansson, S. Discontinuation of low dose aspirin and risk of myocardial infarction: case-control study in UK primary care. *British Medical Journal* 2011; **343**: d4094.
22 Perreault, S., Dragomir, A., Roy, L. et al. Adherence level of antihypertensive agents in coronary artery disease. *British Journal of Clinical Pharmacology* 2010; **69**: 74–84.

2 The mind in medicine

1 Yamazaki, T., Miyazaki, M., Kanase, H., Toyo-Oka, T. and Sugano, K. Transient hypertension in male adolescents when measured by a woman. *Heart* 1998; **79**: 104.
2 Dupre, M.E., George, L.K., Liu, G. and Peterson, E.D. The cumulative effect of unemployment on risks for acute myocardial infarction. *Archives of Internal Medicine* 2012; **172**: 1731–7.
3 O'Keefe, J.H., Carter, M.D. and Lavie, C.J. Primary and secondary prevention of cardiovascular diseases: a practical evidence-based approach. *Mayo Clinic Proceedings* 2009; **84**: 741–57.
4 Uutela, A. Economic crisis and mental health. *Current Opinion in Psychiatry* 2010; **23**: 127–30.
5 Meltzer, H., Bebbington, P., Brugha, T., Farrell, M. and Jenkins, R. The relationship between personal debt and specific common mental disorders. *The European Journal of Public Health* 2013; **23**: 108–13.
6 Loerbroks, A., Apfelbacher, C.J., Thayer, J.F., Debling, D. and Sturmer, T. Neuroticism, extraversion, stressful life events and asthma: a cohort study of middle-aged adults. *Allergy* 2009; **64**: 1444–50.
7 Lala, A., Bobirnac, G. and Tipa, R. Stress levels, alexithymia, type A and type C personality patterns in undergraduate students. *Journal of Medicine and Life* 2010; **3**: 200–5.
8 Denollet, J., Schiffer, A.A. and Spek, V. A general propensity to psychological distress affects cardiovascular outcomes: evidence from research on the type D (distressed) personality profile. *Circulation Cardiovascular Quality and Outcomes* 2010; **3**: 546–57.
9 Tattersall, R. *Diabetes: The biography*. Oxford: Oxford University Press, 2009: 91–2.
10 Morse, D.R., Martin, J. and Moshonov, J. Psychosomatically induced death: relative to stress, hypnosis, mind control, and voodoo: review and possible mechanisms. *Stress Medicine* 1991; **7**: 213–32.
11 Laszlo, K.D., Svensson, T., Li, J. et al. Maternal bereavement during

pregnancy and the risk of stillbirth: a nationwide cohort study in Sweden. *American Journal of Epidemiology* 2013; **177**: 219–27.

12 Dugan, D.O. Laughter and tears: best medicine for stress. *Nursing Forum* 1989; **24**: 18–26.

13 Renzaho, A.M.N., Houng, B., Oldroyd, J., Nicholson, J.M., D'Esposito, F. and Oldenburg, B. Stressful life events and the onset of chronic diseases among Australian adults: findings from a longitudinal survey. *The European Journal of Public Health* 2013, in press.

14 Wall, P.D. Pain and the placebo response. *Ciba Foundation Symposium* 1993; **174**: 187–211; discussion 212–6.

15 Allen, N.B. and Badcock, P.B. Darwinian models of depression: a review of evolutionary accounts of mood and mood disorders. *Progress in Neuro-psychopharmacology & Biological Psychiatry* 2006; **30**: 815–26.

16 Byrne-Davis, L.M.T. and Vedhara, K. Psychoneuroimmunology. *Social and Personality Psychology Compass* 2008; **2**: 751–64.

17 Papac, R.J. Spontaneous regression of cancer. *Cancer Treatment Reviews* 1996; **22**: 395–423.

18 Ventegodt, S., Jacobsen, S. and Merrick, J. Clinical holistic medicine: a case of induced spontaneous remission in a patient with non-Hodgkin b-lymphoma. *Journal of Alternative Medcine Research* 2009; **1**: 101–10.

19 Butow, P.N., Coates, A.S. and Dunn, S.M. Psychosocial predictors of survival: metastatic breast cancer. *Annals of Oncology* 2000; **11**: 469–74.

20 de Craen, A.J., Kaptchuk, T.J., Tijssen, J.G. and Kleijnen, J. Placebos and placebo effects in medicine: historical overview. *Journal of the Royal Society of Medicine* 1999; **92**: 511–15.

21 Vallance, A.K. Something out of nothing: the placebo effect. *Advances in Psychiatric Treatment* 2006; **12**: 287–96.

22 Kemeny, M.E., Rosenwasser, L.J., Panettieri, R.A., Rose, R.M., Berg-Smith, S.M. and Kline, J.N. Placebo response in asthma: a robust and objective phenomenon. *The Journal of Allergy and Clinical Immunology* 2007; **119**: 1375–81.

23 Dorn, S.D., Kaptchuk, T.J., Park, J.B. et al. A meta-analysis of the placebo response in complementary and alternative medicine trials of irritable bowel syndrome. *Neurogastroenterology & Motility* 2007; **19**: 630–7.

24 Emsasi, T., Diener, H., Bussone, G. et al. Placebo-controlled comparison of effervescent acetylsalicylic acid, sumatriptan and ibuprofen in the treatment of migraine attacks. *Cephalalgia* 2004; **24**: 947–54.

25 Huedo-Medina, T.B., Kirsch, I., Middlemass, J., Klonizakis, M. and Siriwardena, A.N. Effectiveness of non-benzodiazepine hypnotics in treatment of adult insomnia: meta-analysis of data submitted to the Food and Drug Administration. *British Medical Journal* 2012; **345**: e8343.

26 Sasannejad, P., Saeedi, M., Shoeibi, A., Gorji, A., Abbasi, M. and Foroughipour, M. Lavender essential oil in the treatment of migraine headache: a placebo-controlled clinical trial. *European Neurology* 2012; **67**: 288–91.

27 Cady, R.K., Goldstein, J., Nett, R., Mitchell, R., Beach, M.E. and Browning, R. A double-blind placebo-controlled pilot study of sublingual feverfew and ginger (LipiGesicTMM) in the treatment of migraine. *Headache: The Journal of Head and Face Pain* 2011; **51**: 1078–86.

28 Greathouse, M. Nebivolol efficacy and safety in patients with stage I–II hypertension. *Clinical Cardiology* 2010; **33**: E20–E7.

29 Cannon, W.B. 'Voodoo' death. *American Anthropologist* 1942; **44**: 169–81.

30 Eastwell, H.D. Voodoo death and the mechanism for dispatch of the dying in East Arnhem, Australia. *American Anthropologist* 1982; **84**: 5–18.

31 Colloca, L. and Miller, F.G. The nocebo effect and its relevance for clinical practice. *Psychosomatic Medicine* 2011; **73**: 598–603.

32 Rief, W., Nestoriuc, Y., von Lilienfeld-Toal, A. et al. Differences in adverse effect reporting in placebo groups in SSRI and tricyclic antidepressant trials: a systematic review and meta-analysis. *Drug Safety* 2009; **32**: 1041–56.

3 The spirit in medicine

1 Mueller, P.S., Plevak, D.J. and Rummans, T.A. Religious involvement, spirituality, and medicine: implications for clinical practice. *Mayo Clinic Proceedings* 2001; **76**: 1225–35.

2 Fingelkurts, A.A. Is our brain hardwired to produce God, or is our brain hardwired to perceive God? A systematic review on the role of the brain in mediating religious experience. *Cognitive Processing* 2009; **10**: 293–326.

3 Vayalilkarottu, J. Holistic health and well-being: a psycho-spiritual/religious and theological perspective. *Asian Journal of Psychiatry* 2012; **5**: 347–50.

4 King, M., Marston, L., McManus, S., Brugha, T., Meltzer, H. and Bebbington, P. Religion, spirituality and mental health: results from a national study of English households. *British Journal of Psychiatry* 2012; **202**: 68–73.

5 Burkhart, L., Schmidt, L. and Hogan, N. Development and psychometric testing of the Spiritual Care Inventory instrument. *Journal of Advanced Nursing* 2011; **67**: 2463–72.

6 McCullough, M.E., Hoyt, W.T., Larson, D.B., Koenig, H.G. and Thoresen, C. Religious involvement and mortality: a meta-analytic review. *Health Psychology* 2000; **19**: 211–22.

7 Reig-Ferrer, A., Arenas, M.D., Ferrer-Cascales, R. et al. Evaluation of spiritual well-being in haemodialysis patients. *Nefrologia : publicacion oficial de la Sociedad Espanola Nefrologia* 2012; **32**: 731–42.

8 Ventegodt, S., Jacobsen, S. and Merrick, J. Clinical holistic medicine: a case of induced spontaneous remission in a patient with non-Hodgkin b-lymphoma. *Journal of Alternative Medicine Research* 2009; **1**: 101–10.

9 Goulding, A. and Ödéhn, N. Schizotypy and mental health in the general population: a pilot study. *Personality and Mental Health* 2009; **3**: 193–202.

10 Robinson, E.A., Krentzman, A.R., Webb, J.R. and Brower, K.J. Six-month changes in spirituality and religiousness in alcoholics predict drinking outcomes at nine months. *Journal of Studies on Alcohol and Drugs* 2011; **72**: 660–8.

11 Vallurupalli, M., Lauderdale, K., Balboni, M.J. et al. The role of spirituality and religious coping in the quality of life of patients with advanced cancer receiving palliative radiation therapy. *Journal of Supportive Oncology* 2012; **10**: 81–7.

12 Delgado-Guay, M.O., Parsons, H.A., Hui, D., de la Cruz, M.G., Thorney, S. and Bruera, E. Spirituality, religiosity, and spiritual pain among caregivers of patients with advanced cancer. *American Journal of Hospice and Palliative Medicine* 2012; **9** (Epub.).

13 Dugan, D.O. Laughter and tears: best medicine for stress. *Nursing Forum* 1989; **24**: 18–26.

14 Park, C.L. and Dornelas, E. Is religious coping related to better quality of life following acute myocardial infarction? *Journal of Religion and Health* 2012; **51**: 1337–46.

15 Gaudia, G. About intercessory prayer: the scientific study of miracles. *Medscape General Medicine* 2007; **9**: 56.

16 Vallance, A.K. Something out of nothing: the placebo effect. *Advances in Psychiatric Treatment* 2006; **12**: 287–96.

17 Wall, P.D. Pain and the placebo response. *Ciba Foundation Symposium* 1993; **174**: 187–211; discussion 212–6.

18 Brown, C.G., Mory, S.C., Williams, R. and McClymond, M.J. Study of the therapeutic effects of proximal intercessory prayer (STEPP) on auditory and visual impairments in rural Mozambique. *Southern Medical Journal* 2010; **103**: 864–9.

19 Byrd, R. Positive therapeutic effects of intercessory prayer in a coronary care unit population. *Southern Medical Journal* 1988; **81**: 826–9.

20 Harris, W.S., Gowda, M., Kolb, J.W., Strychacz, C.P., Vacek, J.L., Jones, P.G., Forker, A., O'Keefe, J.H. and McCallister, B.D. A randomized, controlled trial of the effects of remote, intercessory prayer on outcomes in patients admitted to the coronary care unit. *Archives of Internal Medicine* 1999; **159**: 2273–8.

21 Vannemreddy, P., Bryan, K. and Nanda, A. Influence of prayer and prayer habits on outcome in patients with severe head injury. *American Journal of Hospice and Palliative Medicine* 2009; **26**: 264–9.

22 Lesniak, K.T. The effect of intercessory prayer on wound healing in nonhuman primates. *Alternative Therapies in Health and Medicine* 2006; **12**: 42–8.

23 Sicher, F., Targ, E., Moore, D., II, and Smith, H.S. A randomized double-blind study of the effect of distant healing in a population with

advanced AIDS. Report of a small-scale study. *Western Journal of Medicine* 1998; **169**: 356–63.

24 Astin, J.A., Harkness, E. and Ernst, E. The efficacy of 'distant healing': a systematic review of randomized trials. *Annals of Internal Medicine* 2000; **132**: 903–10.

4 Four steps to help your inner healer

1 Yusuf, S., Hawken, S., Ounpuu, S. et al. Effect of potentially modifiable risk factors associated with myocardial infarction in 52 countries (the INTERHEART study): case-control study. *The Lancet* 2004; **364**: 937–52.

2 Haroon, E., Raison, C.L. and Miller, A.H. Psychoneuroimmunology meets neuropsychopharmacology: translational implications of the impact of inflammation on behavior. *Neuropsychopharmacology* 2012; **37**: 137–62.

3 Rosengren, A., Hawken, S., Ounpuu, S. et al. Association of psychosocial risk factors with risk of acute myocardial infarction in 11 119 cases and 13 648 controls from 52 countries (the INTERHEART study): case-control study. *The Lancet* 2004; **364**: 953–62.

4 Nawrot, T.S., Perez, L., Kunzli, N., Munters, E. and Nemery, B. Public health importance of triggers of myocardial infarction: a comparative risk assessment. *The Lancet* 2011; **377**: 732–40.

5 Richardson, S., Shaffer, J.A., Falzon, L., Krupka, D., Davidson, K.W. and Edmondson, D. Meta-analysis of perceived stress and its association with incident coronary heart disease. *American Journal of Cardiology* 2012; **110**: 1711–16.

6 Lespérance, F., Frasure-Smith, N., Juneau, M. and Théroux, P. Depression and one-year prognosis in unstable angina. *Archives of Internal Medicine* 2000; **160**: 1354–60.

7 Frasure-Smith, N., Lesperance, F. and Talajic, M. Depression following myocardial infarction. Impact on 6-month survival. *JAMA: The Journal of the American Medical Association* 1993; **270**: 1819–25.

8 Vallance, A.K. Something out of nothing: the placebo effect. *Advances in Psychiatric Treatment* 2006; **12**: 287–96.

9 Tsunetsugu, Y., Park, B.-J. and Miyazaki, Y. Trends in research related to 'Shinrin-yoku' (taking in the forest atmosphere or forest bathing) in Japan. *Environmental Health and Preventive Medicine* 2010; **15**: 27–37.

10 Dani, J.A. and Balfour, D.J.K. Historical and current perspective on tobacco use and nicotine addiction. *Trends in Neurosciences* 2011; **34**: 383–92.

11 Pickens, C.L., Airavaara, M., Theberge, F., Fanous, S., Hope, B.T. and Shaham, Y. Neurobiology of the incubation of drug craving. *Trends in Neuroscience* 2011; **34**: 411–20.

12 Hajdu, S.I. A note from history: landmarks in history of cancer, part 3. *Cancer* 2012; **118**: 1155–68.

13 Parkin, D.M. Tobacco-attributable cancer burden in the UK in 2010. *British Journal of Cancer* 2011; **105**: S6–S13.

14 Montgomery, G.H., Schnur, J.B. and Kravits, K. Hypnosis for cancer care: over 200 years young. *CA: A Cancer Journal for Clinicians* 2013; **63**: 31–44.

15 Aubin, H.-J., Farley, A., Lycett, D., Lahmek, P. and Aveyard, P. Weight gain in smokers after quitting cigarettes: meta-analysis. *British Medical Journal* 2012; **345**: e4439.

16 Geary, T., O'Brien, P., Ramsay, S. and Cook, B. A national service evaluation of the impact of alcohol on admissions to Scottish intensive care units. *Anaesthesia* 2012; **67**: 1132–7.

17 Parkin, D.M. and Boyd, L. Cancers attributable to dietary factors in the UK in 2010. *British Journal of Cancer* 2011; **105**: S19–S23.

18 Parkin, D.M. Cancers attributable to consumption of alcohol in the UK in 2010. *British Journal of Cancer* 2011; **105**: S14–S18.

19 Gramenzi, A., Caputo, F., Biselli, M. et al. Review article: alcoholic liver disease – pathophysiological aspects and risk factors. *Alimentary Pharmacology & Therapeutics* 2006; **24**: 1151–61.

20 Seth, D., Haber, P.S., Syn, W.-K., Diehl, A.M. and Day, C.P. Pathogenesis of alcohol-induced liver disease: classical concepts and recent advances. *Journal of Gastroenterology and Hepatology* 2011; **26**: 1089–105.

21 Armstrong, L.E., Ganio, M.S., Casa, D.J. et al. Mild dehydration affects mood in healthy young women. *Journal of Nutrition* 2012; **142**: 382–8.

22 Ganio, M.S., Armstrong, L.E., Casa, D.J. et al. Mild dehydration impairs cognitive performance and mood of men. *British Journal of Nutrition* 2011; **106**: 1535–43.

23 Spigt, M., Weerkamp, N., Troost, J., van Schayck, C.P. and Knottnerus, J.A. A randomized trial on the effects of regular water intake in patients with recurrent headaches. *Family Practice* 2012; **29**: 370–5.

24 Parkin, D.M. and Boyd, L. Cancers attributable to overweight and obesity in the UK in 2010. *British Journal of Cancer* 2011; **105**: S34–S37.

25 Anderson, J.W. and Conley, S.B. Whole grains and diabetes. In: *Whole Grains and Health*. Oxford: Blackwell Publishing Professional, 2007: 29–46.

26 Kromhout, D., Yasuda, S., Geleijnse, J.M. and Shimokawa, H. Fish oil and omega-3 fatty acids in cardiovascular disease: do they really work? *European Heart Journal* 2012; **33**: 436–43.

27 Yokoyama, M., Origasa, H., Matsuzaki, M. et al. Effects of eicosapentaenoic acid on major coronary events in hypercholesterolaemic patients (JELIS): a randomised open-label, blinded endpoint analysis. *The Lancet* 2007; **369**: 1090–8.

28 Toeller, M. Lifestyle issues: diet. In: *Textbook of Diabetes*. Oxford: Wiley-Blackwell, 2010: 346–57.

5 Complementary therapy: supporting your inner healer

1 Park, C. Mind–body CAM interventions: current status and considerations for integration into clinical health psychology. *Journal of Clinical Psychology* 2013; **69**: 45–63.

2 Maggiore, R.J., Gross, C.P., Togawa, K. et al. Use of complementary medications among older adults with cancer. *Cancer* 2012; **118**: 4815–23.

3 Greenfield, S., Pattison, H. and Jolly, K. Use of complementary and alternative medicine and self-tests by coronary heart disease patients. *BMC Complementary and Alternative Medicine* 2008; **8**: 47.

4 Shaw, A., Noble, A., Salisbury, C., Sharp, D., Thompson, E. and Peters, T.J. Predictors of complementary therapy use among asthma patients: results of a primary care survey. *Health & Social Care in the Community* 2008; **16**: 155–64.

5 Thomas, K.J., Nicholl, J.P. and Coleman, P. Use and expenditure on complementary medicine in England: a population based survey. *Complementary Therapies in Medicine* 2001; **9**: 2–11.

6 Vickers, A.J., Cronin, A.M., Maschino, A.C. et al. Acupuncture for chronic pain: individual patient data meta-analysis. *Archives of Internal Medicine* 2012; **172**: 1444–53.

7 Cooley, K., Szczurko, O., Perri, D. et al. Naturopathic care for anxiety: a randomized controlled trial ISRCTN78958974. *PLoS One* 2009; **4**: e6628.

8 The discussion on hypnotism. *British Medical Journal* 1890; **1**: 1259–70.

9 Montgomery, G.H., Schnur, J.B. and Kravits, K. Hypnosis for cancer care: over 200 years young. *CA: A Cancer Journal for Clinicians* 2013; **63**: 31–44.

10 Donesky-Cuenco, D., Nguyen, H.Q., Paul, S. and Carrieri-Kohlman, V. Yoga therapy decreases dyspnea-related distress and improves functional performance in people with chronic obstructive pulmonary disease: a pilot study. *Journal of Alternative and Complementary Medicine* 2009; **15**: 225–34.

11 Cramer, H., Lauche, R., Hohmann, C., Langhorst, J. and Dobos, G. Yoga for chronic neck pain: a 12-month follow-up. *Pain Medicine* 2013; **14**: 541–8.

12 Streeter, C.C., Whitfield, T.H., Owen, L. et al. Effects of yoga versus walking on mood, anxiety, and brain GABA levels: a randomized controlled MRS study. *Journal of Alternative and Complementary Medicine* 2010; **16**: 1145–52.

13 Ross, A., Friedmann, E., Bevans, M. and Thomas, S. Frequency of yoga practice predicts health: results of a national survey of yoga practitioners. *Evidence-based Complementary and Alternative Medicine: eCAM* 2012: 983258.

14 Suarez, A.L., Feramisco, J.D., Koo, J. and Steinhoff, M. Psycho-neuroimmunology of psychological stress and atopic dermatitis: pathophysiologic and therapeutic updates. *Acta Dermato-venereologica* 2012; **92**: 7–15.

15 Goes, T.C., Antunes, F.D., Alves, P.B. and Teixeira-Silva, F. Effect of sweet orange aroma on experimental anxiety in humans. *Journal of Alternative and Complementary Medicine* 2012; **18**: 798–804.

16 Krief, S., Jamart, A., Mahé, S. et al. Clinical and pathologic manifestation of oesophagostomosis in African great apes: does self-medication in wild apes influence disease progression? *Journal of Medical Primatology* 2008; **37**: 188–95.

17 Nibret, E., Ashour, M.L., Rubanza, C.D. and Wink, M. Screening of some Tanzanian medicinal plants for their trypanocidal and cytotoxic activities. *Phytotherapy Research* 2010; **24**: 945–7.

18 Calla-Magarinos, J., Giménez, A., Troye-Blomberg, M. and Fernández, C. An alkaloid extract of Evanta, traditionally used as anti-leishmania agent in Bolivia, inhibits cellular proliferation and interferon-gamma production in polyclonally activated cells. *Scandinavian Journal of Immunology* 2009; **69**: 251–8.

19 Efferth, T. Willmar Schwabe Award 2006: antiplasmodial and antitumor activity of artemisinin – from bench to bedside. *Planta Medica* 2007; **73**: 299–309.

20 Renneberg, R. Biotech history: yew trees, paclitaxel synthesis and fungi. *Biotechnology Journal* 2007; **2**: 1207–9.

21 Sveinsdottir, V., Eriksen, H.R. and Reme, S.E. Assessing the role of cognitive behavioral therapy in the management of chronic nonspecific back pain. *Journal of Pain Research* 2012; **5**: 371–80.

22 Singh, A. Use of mindfulness-based therapies in psychiatry. *Progress in Neurology and Psychiatry* 2012; **16**: 7–11.

23 Rosenkranz, M.A., Davidson, R.J., Maccoon, D.G., Sheridan, J.F., Kalin, N.H. and Lutz, A. A comparison of mindfulness-based stress reduction and an active control in modulation of neurogenic inflammation. *Brain, Behavior, and Immunity* 2013; **27**: 174–84.

24 Itz, C.J., Geurts, J.W., van Kleef, M. and Nelemans, P. Clinical course of non-specific low back pain: a systematic review of prospective cohort studies set in primary care. *European Journal of Pain* 2013; **17**: 5–15.

25 Vidal-Estrada, R., Bosch-Munso, R., Nogueira-Morais, M., Casas-Brugue, M. and Ramos-Quiroga, J.A. Psychological treatment of attention deficit hyperactivity disorder in adults: a systematic review. *Actas espanolas de psiquiatria* 2012; **40**: 147–54.

26 Wiles, N., Thomas, L., Abel, A. et al. Cognitive behavioural therapy as an adjunct to pharmacotherapy for primary care based patients with treatment resistant depression: results of the CoBalT randomised controlled trial. *The Lancet* 2012; **381**: 375–84.

27 Williams, C., Wilson, P., Morrison, J. et al. Guided self-help cognitive behavioural therapy for depression in primary care: a randomised controlled trial. *PLoS One* 2013; **8**: e52735.

6 Your companions for health

1 Germonpré, M., Sablin, M.V., Stevens, R.E. et al. Fossil dogs and wolves from Palaeolithic sites in Belgium, the Ukraine and Russia: osteometry, ancient DNA and stable isotopes. *Journal of Archaeological Science* 2009; **36**: 473–90.

2 Matuszek, S. Animal-facilitated therapy in various patient populations: systematic literature review. *Holistic Nursing Practice* 2010; **24**: 187–203.

3 Charnetski, C.J., Riggers, S. and Brennan, F.X. Effect of petting a dog on immune system function. *Psychological Reports* 2004; **95**: 1087–91.

4 Waite, L.J. and Lehrer, E.L. The benefits from marriage and religion in the United States: a comparative analysis. *Population and Development Review* 2003; **29**: 255–76.

5 Siegler, I.C., Brummett, B.H., Martin, P. and Helms, M.J. Consistency and timing of marital transitions and survival during midlife: the role of personality and health risk behaviors. *Annals of Behavioral Medicine* 2013; **45**: 338–47.

6 King, K.B. and Reis, H.T. Marriage and long-term survival after coronary artery bypass grafting. *Health Psychology* 2012; **31**: 55–62.

7 Ong, A.D., Bergeman, C.S. and Boker, S.M. Resilience comes of age: defining features in later adulthood. *Journal of Personality* 2009; **77**: 1777–804.

8 Kravdal, H. and Syse, A. Changes over time in the effect of marital status on cancer survival. *BMC Public Health* 2011; **11**: 804.

9 Franks, M.M., Stephens, M.A., Rook, K.S., Franklin, B.A., Keteyian, S.J. and Artinian, N.T. Spouses' provision of health-related support and control to patients participating in cardiac rehabilitation. *Journal of Family Psychology* 2006; **20**: 311–18.

10 Kiecolt-Glaser, J.K, Loving, T.J., Stowell, J.R. et al. Hostile marital interactions, proinflammatory cytokine production, and wound healing. *Archives of General Psychiatry* 2005; **62**: 1377–84.

11 Stansfeld, S. and Candy, B. Psychosocial work environment and mental health – a meta-analytic review. *Scandinavian Journal of Work, Environment & Health* 2006; **32**: 443–62.

12 Stansfeld, S.A., Shipley, M.J., Head, J. and Fuhrer, R. Repeated job strain and the risk of depression: longitudinal analyses from the Whitehall II Study. *American Journal of Public Health* 2012; **102**: 2360–6.

7 Resilience and the road to recovery

1 Harvey, S.B., Hatch, S.L., Jones, M. et al. The long-term consequences of military deployment: a 5-year cohort study of United Kingdom reservists deployed to Iraq in 2003. *American Journal of Epidemiology* 2012; **176**: 1177–84.

2 Pedersen, S.S., Kupper, N. and van Domburg, R.T. Heart and mind: are we closer to disentangling the relationship between emotions

and poor prognosis in heart disease? *European Heart Journal* 2011; **32**: 2341–3.

3 Vayalilkarottu, J. Holistic health and well-being: a psycho-spiritual/ religious and theological perspective. *Asian Journal of Psychiatry* 2012; **5**: 347–50.

4 Leamy, M., Bird, V., le Boutillier, C., Williams, J. and Slade, M. Conceptual framework for personal recovery in mental health: systematic review and narrative synthesis. *British Journal of Psychiatry* 2011; **199**: 445–52.

5 Ong, A.D., Bergeman, C.S. and Boker, S.M. Resilience comes of age: defining features in later adulthood. *Journal of Personality* 2009; **77**: 1777–804.

6 Butow, P.N., Coates, A.S. and Dunn, S.M. Psychosocial predictors of survival: metastatic breast cancer. *Annals of Oncology* 2000; **11**: 469–74.

7 Takeda, M., Hashimoto, R., Kudo, T. et al. Laughter and humor as complementary and alternative medicines for dementia patients. *BMC Complementary and Alternative Medicine* 2010; **10**: 28.

8 Dugan, D.O. Laughter and tears: best medicine for stress. *Nursing Forum* 1989; **24**: 18–26.

9 Mora-Ripoll, R. The therapeutic value of laughter in medicine. *Alternative Therapies in Health and Medicine* 2010; **16**: 56–64.

10 Rosengren, A., Hawken, S., Ounpuu, S. et al. Association of psychosocial risk factors with risk of acute myocardial infarction in 11 119 cases and 13 648 controls from 52 countries (the INTERHEART study): case-control study. *The Lancet* 2004; **364**: 953–62.

11 Papac, R.J. Spontaneous regression of cancer. *Cancer Treatment Reviews* 1996; **22**: 395–423.

Further reading

Roberta Bivins, *Alternative Medicine? A history*. Oxford: Oxford University Press, 2007.

David Conway, *The Magic of Herbs*. London: Jonathan Cape, 1973.

Mark Greener, *Which? Way to Manage Your Time – and Your Life*. London: Which? Books, 2000.

Mark Greener, *The Which? Guide to Managing Stress*, second edition. London: Which? Books, 2002.

Mark Greener, *The Heart Attack Survival Guide*. London: Sheldon Press, 2012.

Mark Greener, *Coping with Asthma in Adults*. London: Sheldon Press 2011.

Anne Harrington, *The Cure Within: A history of mind–body medicine*. New York: W.W. Norton, 2008.

Eileen Herzberg, *Thorsons Introductory Guide to Healing*. London: Thorsons, 1988.

Lise Manniche, *An Ancient Egyptian Herbal*. London: British Museum Publications, 1989.

John Polkinghorne, *Exploring Reality*. London: SPCK, 2005.

Andrew Russell, *The Social Basis of Medicine*, first edition. Oxford: Wiley-Blackwell, 2009.

Andrew Scull, *Hysteria: The disturbing history*. Oxford: Oxford University Press, 2011.

Philip Sheldrake, *Spirituality: A very short introduction*. Oxford: Oxford University Press, 2012.

Julia Tugendhat, *How to Approach Death*. London: Sheldon Press, 2007.

Andrew Weil, *Health and Healing: The philosophy of integrative medicine*. London: Warner Books, 1996.

Andrew Weil, *Spontaneous Healing: How to discover and enhance your body's natural ability to maintain and heal itself*. London: Warner Books, 1997.

Charles Wilson, *The Anatomy of Courage*. London: Constable, 2007; first published 1945.

Index